This book is dedicated to my late mom, Gloria Torres, and to my dad and stepmom, Raymond and Nettie DeVallejo. Mom, you taught me the meaning of perseverance. I can feel your presence with me every day; you are my guardian angel. Dad and Nettie, you have instilled in me the importance of having faith in oneself by always having faith in me. I love you with all my heart.

—June Kahn

On the celestial plane, I dedicate this work to the Holy Spirit, for the constant inspiration and unending energy both to and through me. On the human plane of kings and queens, I dedicate this work to Maria Kalofolia, for being a true Hellenic, carpe diem inspiration for early morning cardio workouts. You are a veritable success story.

—Lawrence Biscontini

Morning **Cardio** *Workouts*

June E. Kahn, CPT

Lawrence J.M. Biscontini, MA

Human Kinetics

ALIS

2568666

Library of Congress Cataloging-in-Publication Data

Kahn, June E., 1953-
  Morning cardio workouts / June E. Kahn, Lawrence J.M. Biscontini.
      p. cm.
  Includes bibliographical references and index.
  ISBN-13: 978-0-7360-6369-2 (soft cover)
  ISBN-10: 0-7360-6369-2 (soft cover)
 1. Exercise. 2. Cardiovascular fitness.   I. Biscontini, Lawrence J.M., 1964- II. Title.
  RA781.K234 2007
  613.7'1--dc22

                                           2006026073

ISBN-10: 0-7360-6369-2
ISBN-13: 978-0-7360-6369-2

The Web addresses cited in this text were current as of July 2006, unless otherwise noted.

Acquisitions Editor: Martin Barnard; **Developmental Editor:** Amanda M. Eastin; **Assistant Editor:** Cory Weber; **Copyeditor:** Patsy Fortney; **Proofreader:** Kathy Bennett; **Indexer:** Betty Frizzéll; **Permission Manager:** Carly Breeding; **Graphic Designer:** Bob Reuther; **Graphic Artist:** Tara Welsch; **Photo Managers:** Joe Jovanovich and Brenda Williams; **Cover Designer:** Keith Blomberg; **Photographer (cover):** © Chase Jarvis/Photodisc Royalty-Free; **Photographer (interior):** Tim DeFrisco, unless otherwise noted; **Art Manager:** Kelly Hendren; **Illustrator:** Figures 3.1 and 3.2 by Argosy; figure 3.3 by Mic Greenburg; **Printer:** Sheridan Books

We thank Lakeshore Athletic Club in Broomfield, Colorado, for assistance in providing the location for the photo shoot for this book.

Human Kinetics books are available at special discounts for bulk purchase. Special editions or book excerpts can also be created to specification. For details, contact the Special Sales Manager at Human Kinetics.

Printed in the United States of America   10 9 8 7 6 5 4 3 2 1

Human Kinetics
Web site: www.HumanKinetics.com

United States: Human Kinetics
P.O. Box 5076
Champaign, IL 61825-5076
800-747-4457
e-mail: humank@hkusa.com

Canada: Human Kinetics
475 Devonshire Road Unit 100
Windsor, ON N8Y 2L5
800-465-7301 (in Canada only)
e-mail: orders@hkcanada.com

Europe: Human Kinetics
107 Bradford Road
Stanningley
Leeds LS28 6AT, United Kingdom
+44 (0) 113 255 5665
e-mail: hk@hkeurope.com

Australia: Human Kinetics
57A Price Avenue
Lower Mitcham, South Australia 5062
08 8372 0999
e-mail: liaw@hkaustralia.com

Contents

Preface

If you picked up this book with the hope of getting some new ideas to enhance your existing cardio workouts, then welcome—you have come to the right place and are about to embark on a journey that will give you everything you need, and more! *Morning Cardio Workouts* targets the needs of dedicated fitness enthusiasts looking for options for their morning cardio workout. But it doesn't end there.

Having instructed fitness professionals and fitness enthusiasts for over a combined 50 years, we, June and Lawrence, are dedicated cardio enthusiasts ourselves. We understand the need to find ways to vary our routines. We appreciate the fun; the challenge; and the need for creative, exciting, and varied cardio workouts. We have done everything from fun runs to ocean jogging, from Hollywood hiking to stroller pushing, from deep-water running to indoor cycling sprints. We have climbed mountains and taught step classes. Yep, we've done it all. We have trained alone, in groups, with teams, and with partners (and discovered that some workouts are far less exciting than others!). Between us, we've appeared on *CNN Headline News*, *Good Morning America*, *LIVE with Regis and Kelly*, and the QVC network; served as fitness consultant for the soap opera *General Hospital*; starred in a variety of fitness instructor training videos; and traveled the globe teaching cutting-edge fitness techniques—we are the experts who train the trainers, and it is with this wealth of experience and success with cardiovascular workout programs that we present this book to you. We know how to work it in and work it out!

There are many reasons for incorporating cardio workouts into your morning routine. If you are already involved in a regular morning cardio routine, maybe you are looking for new ideas to cross-train and add variety to your workouts. If your goal is to lose weight, then maybe you have chosen the activity because you have heard that it burns the most calories. Perhaps your physician has suggested that you start a cardio program to improve your health. Or maybe you choose to involve yourself in a cardio workout because you find it reduces your stress level. Whatever your reason or personal goals, *Morning Cardio Workouts* will provide you with all the tools, mental preparation, and information (including the latest in cutting-edge fitness research) you need to get the most out of your workout.

The benefits of regular morning cardio workouts are many. To start, you get a great deal of fitness work done and over with early in the day. Oftentimes, putting off the cardio workout until the end of the day means that you find yourself tired in the afternoon or evening and, consequently, skip the cardiovascular workout totally. The early morning cardio workout, however, will help you avoid that scenario. Also, once you tax your heart beyond its normal function, many physical benefits ensue, not the least of which can be a heightened sense of energy for the remainder of the day. A morning cardio workout can also improve digestion for the rest of the day, improve alertness, help your body become more efficient with daily tasks so that you invest less energy to accomplish the same amount of work, assist with general function improvement in daily tasks, increase your heart pump's efficiency (stroke volume) and cardiac output (volume per minute), increase your body's ability to extract oxygen from the blood, reduce the risk of premature heart attack and stroke, decrease body weight and body fat, improve bone density, improve blood glucose control, improve psychological and physical well-being, improve sleep quality, and even increase life expectancy (American College of Sports Medicine 1998).

But the benefits of morning exercise don't stop there. This book is unique in that it is not just about the physical benefits for the body; it is also about the benefits to the person as a whole: body, mind, and spirit. *Morning Cardio Workouts* tells you how to get the best cardio workout for *you*.

By learning how to embrace and incorporate the concept of mindfulness using our brain–body–breath approach, you will learn how to commit to the workout *and* yourself with a mindful approach to exercise that not only maximizes physical benefits but also crosses over to every aspect of your life. You literally train from the inside out using your inner connected self to improve the outer you! We also reinforce our workouts and ideas with the motto *carpe diem*, which is Latin for "seize the day." This motto will keep you focused on the present and on making each day and each workout count.

Morning Cardio Workouts is divided into two parts. Part one addresses your a.m. readiness, for complete preparation in all aspects of your workout including energy requirements, rest, and sleep considerations. We also explore mind–body awareness, our holistic approach to fitness that incorporates the brain–body–breath connection. You will find complete descriptions of and information on a variety of cardio activities for both outside and inside as well as group exercise options. In addition, we take you on a tour of how the muscles in the body respond and develop to the training and overload that your morning cardio workout provides, including proper warm-up and injury prevention techniques.

Part two has something for everybody. It focuses on intensity choices ranging from light-effort workouts to high-effort workouts that are separated into specific time frames so you can choose the time that will fit the best into your already packed morning schedule. We also include ideas for a variety of recovery workouts. In all this information and more on disciplines that will enhance and balance your workouts as well as your daily life, you can't help but find something that you love in the workouts found in this book.

We're confident that you will leave this text with options and information galore no matter what your body type, fitness level, or workout preferences. Now is the time to start creating your own personal success story. *Carpe diem!*

Acknowledgments

They say that success comes from the support of family, friends, and colleagues along the way—and from unconditional faith in oneself. This was truly the case in the process of putting this book together. I have dedicated my life and career to educating people in the ways to enhance their lifestyles through proper exercise. It is a passion I have fulfilled by traveling and sharing with many people along the way. However, sitting down and putting things in writing was not an easy process for me. It required the collaboration of many people who helped me in so many ways, and I would like to take the time to thank them. Without their input and support, this project could never have been accomplished.

I want to thank Sara Kooperman for pulling me into this project in the first place, but more for her guidance, support, friendship, and faith in me over the years.

Lawrence, my dear friend and colleague, for coming through for me, time and time again, even with his overseas ventures, and for his valuable contributions and insights as my coauthor.

Martin Barnard, senior acquisitions editor at Human Kinetics, for having the faith in me to complete this project, and giving me this incredible opportunity. I want to thank him for his patience, but most of all for his support. Mandy Eastin, our editor at Human Kinetics, for her energy, consistent support, understanding, and valuable input, and for always keeping me on task.

Len Kravitz, for his research contributions. Kerri Salazar, my talented assistant, who helped compile research, edited, and was invaluable in the workout creation sections. I could not have completed this without her help. Shannon Griffiths, my colleague and friend, for her input and incredible support during the lengthy process of putting this together—she has enhanced my attention to detail. Thank you, Shannon, for always being there.

Cameron Chinatti, for her input in the workout creation, and for her insight and creativity. Lakeshore Athletic Club, for allowing us to use their wonderful facility as a backdrop to our photo shoot. Linda Shelton, for her mentorship and advice on overcoming writer's block! Our models—Thea Thompson, Dee Ackerman, and Shanley McClure—for their enthusiasm and great bodies! Thomas Donia for his support and assistance in gathering up the equipment necessary for our photoshoot. And finally, Jim Hussey, for always helping me see the bigger picture throughout the final process, which gave me invaluable consumer insight—you inspired me. My heart has been touched with enormous gratitude to all of these people—more than I can ever express in a few sentences here. This project could not have come to completion without them.

—June Kahn

No product of the *present* is possible without a fused process of the *past*. With gratitude, I acknowledge those people who have inspired me in some way that directly or indirectly made my ideas in this book possible.

I thank June Kahn, who invited me to coauthor this labor of love with her so long ago.

I humbly thank God for infinite blessings, inspiration, and energy, and Constance Mary Towers, the apotheosis of impromptu grace and elocution (for her unending understanding, eloquence, and positivism). I know her support of *Morning Cardio Workouts* began at the start, and for that I am grateful. She truly is covered with the fingerprints of God.

I also thank Alana (for the "support and Scrabbles" during the 2005 Mykonian season when I wrote this book); Maria Gavin; Sara Kooperman (for the Mania madness); Petra Kolber (for the professional advice); C Mark Rees (for FG2000); the entire Golden Door Puerto Rico team (for constant support both at my position and away from it); Stephanie Montgomery at Reebok; AFAA (especially Laurie and Lisa); ACE (especially Stacey, Kristie, and Brian); AEA (Julie and Angie); the AFPP (especially Tina Juan, Shirley, and Bam!); Mike and Stephanie Morris (for the teamwork on the BALL); Len Kravitz (for the mentoring and research); the gals at John and Ankie's Bodywork Gym in Mykonos, who had more of an open mind to everything than I ever thought possible; Diane Berson and J Sklar (for the details); Susan L. Fischer (for transcendence in education); Tom Snow (for the original "Yo-Chi" music for those early mind-body walks); Robert Milazzo (for the photos); the Xerox Queen herself, Maria Kalofolia (for the truest friendship); Ankie and John (for the Bodywork Gym hours); Kathie and Peter Davis for IDEA; Maureen Hagan for the Canadian fun at CanFitPro; Carol for ECA; Bernard Hasse (for the Hasenhau); Irene "Cathy" Narvaez (for the hundreds of e-mails as a premium personal assistant); Liz Kalmanowicz (for keeping the money flowing); all of the colleagues who have come to any fitness session of mine at any convention anywhere; and Barbara.

—Lawrence Biscontini

A.M. Readiness

The format of our book is simple. We want you to set realistic goals, maximize the benefits you want, and minimize the amount of time needed to achieve your goals. Part one gets you started. Chapters 1 through 6 give you the background information you need to get ready. In chapter 1 you will find information ranging from fueling your body to keeping yourself motivated on those mornings you would rather just turn the alarm off, roll over, and go back to sleep. Chapter 2 is about you. It helps you take an internal look at yourself and find ways to set your workout goals, track your workouts, and "seize your day!" Chapter 3 offers an overview of your muscles, leaving you with an understanding of what it takes for the major muscles of your body to power your workouts, including the most important muscle of all, your heart! Chapters 4, 5, and 6 offer outdoor, indoor, and group activity options. In these chapters you will learn what the activities are all about, what muscles benefit, and technique tips for how to do the activities the most efficiently and effectively. This is all great information to prepare you in body and mind for part two—the workouts!

In this book we are addressing men and women who enjoy getting the most out of each morning workout, who are looking for diversity in their routines, and who are not new to fitness. However, we welcome anyone to begin a new fitness program at any time with proper medical clearance. You will find two overall approaches to fitness in this book: (1) great ideas to maintain your fitness level, and (2) exciting ways to improve it. Before starting any fitness program, the most important prerequisite is medical approval. Especially if you are over the age of 55, make sure you have a specific discussion with your medical care practitioner (American Council on Exercise 2004; Gladwin 2003). We also assume that you are open to new ideas. Because current research shows that the best way to improve your fitness level is not to undertake a single activity but to incorporate change itself into your program, we offer a plethora of ideas to help put variation into your routines (Kravitz 1994).

Our first premise is deceptively simple: If nothing changes, nothing changes. This book will give you ideas on how to change your early morning cardiovascular work with a strong attention to mindfulness. You've purchased this book because you want change. The exerciser who wants to improve her fitness, but who does little to change her routine may end up wondering why she is seeing so few benefits and changes. If your routine doesn't change periodically, your body won't change either.

Because we believe so strongly in changing your early morning cardiovascular workouts, we give you a wide variety of specific workouts in part two of this book. Enter June and Lawrence to take you through a world of options to maximize this change, all while respecting your time. We've compiled specific workouts with both specific and general guidelines. Just choose options that will work for you! Throughout this book we refer to these changes as ways to tax the cardiovascular system, which means to impose demands on your heart and other systems of your body to make them work more intensely than they do during your everyday functions at work, play, or repose.

Finally, the best news is that you cannot fail with this book. There is no pass or fail to any suggested routine or program. We provide options and ideas for you to get the most out of your routine, knowing that no written path is a path for everyone. Trust your instincts. Stay open to that little voice that tells you what is working. Omit what is not. *Most importantly, remember that as long as you are moving in some capacity, you are moving toward success!*

1

Energy to Start the Day

||||||||||||||||||||||||||||||||||||||||||||||||||||||||||||||||||||||||||||||||||||||||||||||||||||||||||||||||||||||||||||||

Working out in the early morning helps you seize the day to capture a multitude of benefits. The ancient Romans used the Latin term *carpe diem* to signify accomplishing the bulk of necessary work and pleasure before noontime. Afterward, time was dedicated to eating long meals throughout the afternoon, followed by generous portions of sleep. Late afternoons were for work, followed by supper and bed. Our book draws on the premise of carpe diem as well in an effort to show you the benefits of working out in the early morning. Not only will you get your physical exercise out of the way first thing in the morning, but you can enjoy the benefits all during your day: increased alertness, a greater sense of vitality, a feeling of mind–body connectedness, more energy to get things done, and an increase in overall well-being for the day. This chapter outlines how to maximize your energy in the morning so you can start your morning workouts right.

Sleep

Because you will be engaging in your morning cardio workout after a night of sleep, a brief discussion of sleep will help you understand its purpose. During sleep, the body repairs and heals itself from all of the work it has performed during the day. At the cellular and muscular levels, rest allows cells and muscles to return to a state of homeostasis, which means, among other things, a balanced alkaline/acidity level. During sleep, the heart rate lowers, which allows the other systems of the body such as the digestive and circulatory systems to rest and repair as well. These systems don't stop working; they just slow down to recover from their more active roles during the day when you are moving and digesting.

Optimizing your sleep is important to feeling your best during your morning workout. When you miss out on sleep, try to recover the time you missed on the next available sleep time. Current research states that adults should get a minimum of between eight and nine hours of sleep per night for rest and repair. Because achieving deep states of sleep is important for your body to rest and repair, and because you will be asking your body to work hard in the early morning, you should speak with your medical care practitioner if you are not achieving a high quality of sleep for any extended period.

There are some things you can control to optimize sleep. Comfortable, natural fiber clothing allows your skin to breathe while you sleep. Adequate bedding provides proper ventilation and added comfort. A pillow that is best for your posture and breathing (soft or hard, hypoallergenic) can help you sleep more deeply. Finally, the quieter your environment is, the deeper you will sleep, so try to minimize distractions around your sleeping area.

Learn to listen to your body. If you feel sluggish and tired, instead of asking your body to perform a vigorous morning cardio workout, refer to one of our recovery workouts in chapter 10. Working out hard can be dangerous if you are overtired because, not only will you not be able to perform to the levels of intensity you wish, but you will also be more prone to injury.

Nutrition

Proper nutrition means giving your body the necessary fuel to perform. Think of your body as a fine-tuned piece of valuable machinery, such as a car. Nobody would expect to make demands of a wonderfully strong vehicle with an empty gas tank. Likewise, before asking your body to work hard for you, you should provide it with fuel, one of the most important prerequisites for cardiovascular exercise.

Fuel for the body first and foremost means food. The body cannot function without food, and specific to morning workouts, this means breakfast. We've mentioned that most people need at least eight hours of sleep per night, and this means that everyone wakes up in a relative state of hypoglycemia, or low blood sugar. Before working out, therefore, you have low blood sugar because you probably haven't eaten for eight hours of sleep plus the hours between your last meal and sleep. If you eat finish dinner at 7 p.m., go to bed at 10 p.m., and wake up at 6 a.m., your blood sugar is low because you haven't had any caloric nutrition for 11 hours! You must ingest enough calories to offset this because (1) your body needs to return to an elevated level of blood sugar for normal function and (2) your body is about to endure an intensive caloric expenditure. Among the benefits of eating before working out are returning your body to a normal blood sugar level and giving yourself the additional calories you need to jump-start your engine for the workout. Nobody should run on empty, quite literally, because the body will have to turn to its own stores of glycogen (carbohydrate calories) for fuel, and this storage is meant for emergencies, not for normal exercise.

We do not recommend engaging in any early morning cardio workout on an empty stomach, with the body in a hypoglycemic state. Choose how heavy your breakfast will be based on how heavy your chosen intensity will be for any given workout for that day. The more calories you ingest, the longer you usually need to wait before an intense workout. A full English breakfast, for example (eggs, bacon, sausages, beans on toast, croissant, tea, scones, and jam), before a run may be contraindicated. Eating a part of that before the run would yield a more comfortable run. As soon as you finish the run, you can finish the breakfast.

There is no one set breakfast for everyone to maximize energy, but you can choose from various combinations of carbohydrate, protein, and fat to jump-start your day. Leading sport nutritionists tell us that the bulk of our calories, about 55 to 60 percent, should ideally come from complex carbohydrates, followed by 10 to 15 percent from a combination of lean proteins, and up to 30 percent from Mediterranean-style fats such as olive oil, nut oils (e.g., almond or walnut), avocados, and fish oils (McArdle, Katch, Katch 1998). This recommended percentage optimizes the way the body digests food and turns it into energy (called ATP) for the longest period of time. Not achieving a balanced ratio will produce less-than-ideal results. For example, a snack or meal too high in carbohydrates with no fat and protein combination will give an instant feeling of fullness, but quickly into the workout you will "crash" or "hit the wall" and feel energy depleted. Table 1.1 shows some possible combinations of carbohydrates, proteins, and fats. Bear in mind that these combinations are offered for illustrative purposes and by no means should serve as a meal plan for every person.

When your morning cardio workout will be particularly intense and would preclude you from having a full, healthful breakfast immediately preceding your workout, be sure to have at least *some* combination of carbohydrate, fat, and protein before starting (e.g., half a whole wheat bagel with 2 teaspoons [about 1 ml] of peanut butter and 8 ounces [227 g] of water, or a soy or yogurt–fruit-juice drink).

Regardless of how many calories you choose to ingest, and regardless of the intensity of your workout, remember that for proper hydration there is no substitute for ample amounts of water before a workout (see the hydration section for more information). A complete breakfast should then follow the workout, meaning that you should take nourishment before 60 minutes have gone by to avoid the risk of low blood sugar.

Table 1.1 **Sample Balanced-Ratio Meals**

Combination	Carbohydrates	Fats	Proteins	Breakdown
1 (approximately 250 calories)	1 cup cooked oatmeal topped with 2 tsp. honey	1/4 cup almonds	2 egg whites	55% carb, 25% fat, and 20% protein
2 (approximately 250 calories)	1 cup low-fat yogurt with fruit; 2 slices whole wheat toast	1 tbsp. peanut butter	Yogurt, bread, and peanut butter	55% carb, 25% fat, and 20% protein
3 (approximately 425 calories)	2 whole wheat pancakes (prepared with skim milk and 2 egg whites) topped with 2 tsp. honey; 1/2 cup yogurt; 1/2 cup raisins	1 tsp. trans fat-free margarine; 1 tsp. olive oil	Egg whites, flour, and yogurt	55% carb, 25% fat, and 20% protein
4 (approximately 450 calories)	Fresh fruit smoothie (made with 1 kiwi, 1 orange, 1 banana, 1 apple [with skin], 1 dash cinnamon, and 1 dash mace)	1 tbsp. almonds or walnuts	2% milk (or light soy milk) with 1 scoop of whey protein powder	60% card, 20% fat, and 20% protein

A car must have gasoline in its engine to perform work, but the engine can use the gas only if it has appropriate amounts of motor oil. The equivalent of motor oil in the human body is three things: water, vitamins, and minerals. Without these three things, the body cannot perform work efficiently and achieve desired results. Because hydration is such a hot topic in exercise, water is discussed separately in the next section. The vitamins and minerals that make up the other part of the motor oil for the human engine are called micronutrients. If we plan our meals using the newly revised guidelines of the USDA Food Guide Pyramid, we should absorb enough vitamins and nutrients from our food that we do not need to ingest them as supplements.

People who cannot find appropriate choices of food in appropriate quantities (those who travel frequently, for example) may be helped by vitamins and minerals supplements. Because of the extreme personal nature of supplements and individual physiology, we don't recommend the supplementation of vitamins or minerals without the supervision of a medical care provider. The market offers a plethora of options, and as such, only your medical care provider knows enough about your complete profile to be able to recommend what you need to supplement—if anything—based on your health history and detailed blood profiles performed during annual physical examinations.

Hydration

Every living organism needs water, and lots of it. The ancient root word *aquam* not only signified water, but also life. Today, spas around the world draw on this association of water with life. The word *spa*, incidentally, comes from the complete Latin phrase *solus per aquam*, or "complete wellness from water." Although the presence of water in the body does not guarantee health, it most definitely is the first building block of proper body function and maintenance.

Water is a macronutrient. This means you have to ingest it often because it's so necessary for life. Water fills cells with necessary liquid so they can complete their functions of producing energy and carrying waste products from the body. Water also makes up 80 percent of muscle and 60 percent of the body. Water keeps the skin healthy, the organs fed with blood and nutrients, and the brain functioning, among other things. We recommend drinking enough water so that you are never thirsty and so that urine is always clear and copious. Although we are a highly evolved species, our thirst mechanism lags behind our need for water. This means that when you are thirsty, your body is usually past the point of needing water and starting to dehydrate. Remember to drink enough water so your urine is clear. Other drinks do not count as water because they contain other ingredients that can negate water's absorption, such as caffeine. Research shows that cool water (not frozen) absorbs faster from the stomach than warm water, so our recommendation for hydration is cool water (American Council on Exercise 2004).

If the purpose of your morning cardio workout is weight maintenance or weight reduction, we do not recommend replacement sport drinks for hydration during cardiovascular events under 60 minutes long (Yorke 2001). The reason is, quite simply, that you would be consuming the very calories you are trying to burn off. For example, if you are running on a treadmill for 50 minutes (burning approximately 200 calories) and simultaneously sipping on a sport drink (ingesting approximately 200 calories), you could be undermining your goal of weight loss. During the workout, water is a more logical choice because it hydrates the body without adding unnecessary calories. When your cardiovascular workout exceeds 60 minutes, such as in an endurance run or marathon, then the experts recommend ingesting additional calories because you are already burning off more than you are consuming.

Because hydration is important before, after, and during cardiovascular workouts, being able to carry water is a plus if this is possible for you. Many companies

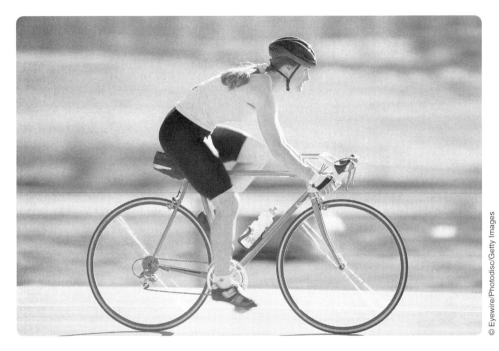

© Eyewire/Photodisc/Getty Images

Take a water bottle with you to ensure you stay hydrated during your morning workouts.

make water bottles now that attach to belt loops, strap across the back, and even fit into hats, to make hydration easy and convenient during cardiovascular events. Choose whatever works for you that allows you to stay hydrated in all types of weather and during all types of events.

Because we are discussing the importance of breakfast in the early morning workout, and because breakfast often includes coffee or tea, we now turn to a current hot topic: caffeine. In most of the world, caffeine is a legalized drug, or stimulant. Although this is a highly debated issue, current research reveals that small amounts of caffeine (Dodd, Herb, and Powers 1993) (the equivalent of about 1/2 cup [113 g] of coffee or 1/2 can [170 g] of soda with caffeine) before cardiovascular workouts can help free up additional fat cells from adipose tissue with greater ease for a slightly higher burn of fat during that exercise bout. Caffeine makes the adrenal glands produce epinephrine and norepinephrine, which makes the body feel more powerful and energetic. Because caffeine arouses the central nervous system, it increases the availability of fatty acids and delays muscle fatigue in endurance performance activities such as running.

Unfortunately, many people interpret this quality of caffeine to mean "the more caffeine I drink, the more fat I will burn," which simply is not the case. Too much caffeine robs the muscles of the water they need to perform. As the body loses water, breakdown commences at the cellular level. Furthermore, too much caffeine can overwork the kidneys; lead to insomnia, heart arrhythmias, and other cardiac irregularities; produce restlessness; and be psychologically addicting. We don't endorse the drinking of caffeine before your morning cardio workouts without consulting with your medical care practitioner. Only he or she understands your complete health profile and can predict any possible interactions caffeine may have with other supplements and any prescribed medication you may be taking. Even if you are taking something as apparently innocuous as aspirin, for example, your doctor should know about caffeine usage because of the potentially hazardous combination of these two substances.

Clothing and Footwear

Although it's been said that clothes make the man or woman, it is also true that the right choice of clothing can "make the workout." This means that choosing the appropriate material and combination of items can improve your body's efficacy. After breakfast and hydrating, be sure to spend some time choosing your apparel carefully. Beginning with your foundation, your feet, choose footwear that's appropriate for your specific tasks. Cross-training shoes with appropriate ankle support improve safety. For running on uneven outdoor terrain, shoes with improved undersole traction are necessary. If running is your mode of choice, you will be thankful for choosing lighter-weight shoes. Be sure to put your shoes on carefully, lacing up from the part of the shoe closest to the toes and finishing with tying the laces. Many people put on and remove their fitness shoes without taking the time to lace up and lace down appropriately, causing a stretched-out upper-shoe tongue that does little to support the foot during the workout. Above all, a shoe that feels comfortable with enough lateral support and cushioning is a must.

Consider wind chill, altitude, heat, and humidity when choosing your fitness apparel. Clothing made from new fabrics that pull sweat away from the body immediately prove highly comfortable, allowing the body to work efficiently in hot and humid conditions. If wind chill is a factor, a light outer jacket may also be necessary to provide an additional layer of warmth between you and the wind. If you are engaging in your morning cardio workout at high altitude, dressing in layers may be necessary because you may fatigue, slow down, and consequently become colder and need to put on a layer of clothing for warmth. Depending on your geographic area and the temperature in the early morning, dressing in layers will help the body thermoregulate as it changes its intensity during warm-up, work, and transition phases of the workout. A lightweight jacket that you can take off easily and tie around your waist can be a comfortable addition to your wardrobe.

Clothing that stays put while allowing movement will be the most comfortable during your workout. In this book we emphasize the breath in our brain–body–breath connection. Because the breath is essential to the workout, be sure to avoid clothing that restricts the waistline because this could impair breathing. Anything with a tight waistband (even elastic can be too tight) will restrict the movement of your diaphragm during your workout when you start breathing harder.

Clothes that move too much around the body, such as pants or shorts that "crawl" down the body as you begin to move quickly, very soon prove distracting. Depending on how early your workout will be, there may be no sun to illuminate your way. Brightly colored clothing designed for runners reflects headlights, thereby serving an additional safety function.

If your morning cardio workout involves the aquatic environment, choose a bathing suit that makes you feel the most comfortable and mobile. New synthetic fabrics that are quick drying may prove important if you are not changing after your workout such as when on a beach or at a resort pool. Be aware that most swimming environments now mandate swimming caps for men and women, so you may want to budget this into your initial expense.

Hats have a variety of purposes: shielding the eyes from the sun, holding down hair, serving as reflectors for traffic, and making a fashion statement, among others. Because the head is a major escape route for heat during exercise, putting on a solid hat can be like putting a lid on a rapidly boiling pot of water. Depending on the intensity of your cardio workout and the temperature, a cap could affect your body's ability to thermoregulate appropriately by preventing heat escape. If you choose a cap, therefore, choose one that allows heat to escape easily, such as one made of mesh or a light fabric. Finally, checking the local weather report before any outdoor workout will help you choose the appropriate amount of layers, reflective clothing, and any needed waterproof materials you may need to enhance your safety, movement, and comfort.

Music motivates many of us, and recent research has shown that adding music to a workout actually can help burn calories (Biley 2000). To be sure, safety is the first issue, so be sure that the headphones of your CD player, MP3 player, or other portable music device stay secure during movement—yet another use for a hat! To stay safe, remember to keep the volume of your music low because you must be able to hear important surrounding noises, such as telephones and doorbells inside, and car horns and wildlife outside. Choose music that motivates you to put more energy into your workout for an increased energy expenditure.

If you understand beats per minute and like to move with the music, you may want to choose music speed that most appropriately complements your moves, such as music that has beats that most closely match the pace at which you run. An ample selection of professionally mixed music is available for fitness enthusiasts such as steppers, runners, and even those who kayak at a certain pace. From companies such as Dynamix Music, for example, you just have to choose the genre of music you like (e.g., top radio hits, country, or oldies) and the pace of the music you like, which is referred to in terms of beats per minute. Typical beats per minute for stepping-like activities or slow walking are around 130 beats per minute, whereas runners may choose faster-paced music from 140 to 150 beats per minute.

Appropriate music can boost your motivation and energy level, your caloric expenditure, and your overall enjoyment of your morning cardio workout. So if you want to work out to music, don't forget your headphones when planning your wardrobe.

Recovery

Recovery refers to the time it takes for the body to heal itself after a workout. This can be in the form of sleep (discussed earlier in the chapter) or rest. There are two types of rest. The first is simply doing nothing. The second is called active recovery and is discussed in detail in chapter 10.

For the purposes of this book, we define rest as time away from working out. Oftentimes, we can get carried away by the new feelings of endorphins that our new routines bring. Endorphins in the brain make us feel energized, euphoric, and even stronger. Sometimes we are tempted to exercise even more because these endorphin chemicals can almost be addicting. To avoid burnout and muscle overuse, and to allow proper time for muscles to recover and rest between workouts, the body needs rest. Remembering to *rest and recover as intensively as you train* will help you stay focused on a balanced program that involves taxing the cardiovascular system and then letting it recover. Although some people think that the body stops burning calories after a workout, the truth is that a fit person burns more calories at rest than an inactive person, even during recovery for up to two hours after a workout, especially when the activity session has lasted at least 30 minutes (Kravitz 1994; Wilmore and Costill 1990).

Another definition of recovery has to do with the muscles themselves. When we tax the different systems of the body when we run, for example, small damages occur to the skeletal muscles (such as the gastrocnemius, or calf muscle). These small damages are normal, and the body repairs them efficiently and quickly. This occurs only during rest, however. Engaging in a morning cardio workout every day can be safe. Learn to listen to your body, however. If you feel sickly or weak, it may be best to avoid exercise until you start to feel more normal. Avoiding rest by engaging in too many intensely sequenced bouts of exercise will keep these muscular restorations from occurring, leaving the muscles open to damage. Possible results can be muscle injuries such as sprains and strains and an increased resting heart rate. Finally, women should know that another symptom of overtraining and not giving the body adequate time to repair itself can be the temporary loss of the monthly menstrual cycle.

Taxing the same muscles in the same way every day can lead to injury. This book offers a wide variety of workouts so that you don't encounter that situation. For example, one day you may choose a workout involving a weight-bearing activity such as running, and on the next day you may choose something that minimizes the taxation to the lower legs, such as an aquatic workout or a workout on a recumbent bicycle. Remember to rest as often as you work out to maximize your workouts. Instead of thinking you are taking it easy, think of it instead as giving your engine a tune-up in the shop so it can efficiently, energetically, and productively work for you again.

In short, as you prepare for your morning cardio workout, remember the prerequisites to maximizing your results: a proper breakfast, hydration, and rest. If you are missing one or more of these prerequisites, it may be best to either abstain from exercising until you can meet these bare requirements or to choose a much lower intensity than normal. Your body will thank you, and your workout will be more productive when you do.

Motivation

Even though you are—or soon will be—a dedicated morning exerciser (hey, you bought this book!), we acknowledge that everyone has the occasional day of feeling unmotivated. Here are some tips to get you out of this possible slump.

Although choosing a morning cardio workout is an individual decision, remember that not all training has to be a solitary experience. Once you have established realistic goals (see chapter 2 for information on goal setting), consider the fact that other people, those who are part of and those who are adjacent to your social circle, can influence the attainment of your goals. To be sure, you can choose to work out alone with almost any of the workouts detailed in this book. But social support can provide extra motivation to succeed with your program.

Motivation can be either internal (coming from yourself) or external (coming from others). Staying motivated means maintaining an honest awareness of your feelings while periodically checking your goals as constant reminders of *why* you are working out. When you begin a fitness program, we suggest that you make a list (see chapter 2 for details) of both internal and external rewards that come from your workouts. Internal rewards and goals come from feelings and measurable changes that come from inside, such as *feeling* happier and *measuring* smaller at the waistline or larger at the triceps. External rewards come from people and situations and can include such things as compliments from others when you look fitter, and noticing how the airplane seatbelt fits around you.

The following suggestions may help you motivate yourself when you know you should engage in a morning cardio workout but do not quite feel motivated:

- Review both the intrinsic and extrinsic goals that you've written down or typed out.
- Remind yourself of the long-term health benefits occurring as a direct result of your workout.
- Remember the endorphins that will be released after you start exercising. These chemicals can motivate you further because they give you a sense of well-being. These include serotonin, a chemical released between your brain cells that makes you feel happy. This can be a healthy addiction: The more you want to feel good, the more you will be motivated to exercise!
- Try to imagine your body closer to your realistic goals as a direct result of the ensuing workout.
- Find your most motivating music to listen to during your workout, if appropriate.
- Engage in positive self-talk when facing yourself in the bathroom by looking right into your own eyes and telling yourself out loud, "I am going to give myself a fantastic workout this morning because I am worth it." Even if you do not quite feel up to such a workout, remembering the adage "fake it until you make it" can help greatly.

External motivation, such as extrinsic goals, comes from others. In some instances, friends and family members can offer support. If appropriate, look to family members and friends for help by doing the following:

- Invite a family member or friend to work out with you.
- Ask a family member or friend to wake you up with an encouraging, motivating telephone call early in the morning before your workout.
- Ask a family member or friend to verbalize positive changes they observe in both your personality and your physical body.

The smaller, more personalized partnership of just one person also can offer motivation. Choosing a workout partner who can participate in your morning cardio workouts almost every time that you do can bring more specific and individualized motivation. When you have a consistent workout partner, you can rely on him or her more strongly than you can on a group for the following:

- Motivating telephone calls
- Pep talks when you aren't quite up to working out
- Positive comments about what he or she notices in you, such as increased energy, endurance, intensity, and weight loss
- Encouraging e-mails
- Exciting conversation during your morning cardio workouts, if appropriate

If you are part of a partnership, make sure you have proper partner etiquette. Good workout partner etiquette includes the following actions:

- **Being specific when giving feedback.** Instead of saying, "You're looking great today," for example, a helpful partner can offer a more specific comment such as, "Those same pants looked tighter on you last month" or "You've got such an energetic smile today." Observable, measurable feedback using a tangible reference point seems more sincere than a general comment.
- **Asking open-ended questions.** Instead of asking a question that can be answered with a yes or no, a partner can ask an open-ended question that invites discussion; this can lead to more motivating conversation. Instead of asking, "Do you feel like working out this morning?" asking "How do you feel about working out this morning?" will invite more conversation.
- **Providing encouraging motivation from time to time.** The occasional voice or text message sent to a mobile telephone, answering machine, or e-mail account can let your partner know that you are motivated about the morning cardio workout and anticipating the next one. In this way, motivation can be contagious.

Group exercise classes offer the motivation benefits of group dynamics without giving you the added task of having to search out a group. Any group fitness instructor will tell you that microsocieties form in clubs among the participants

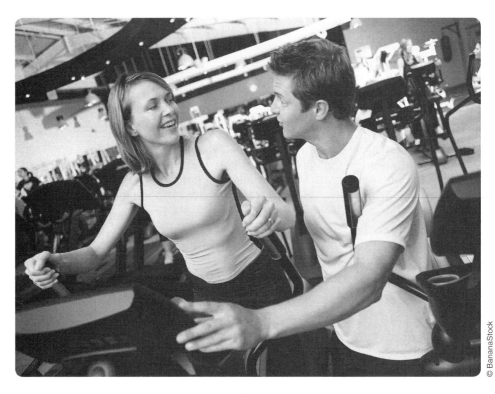

© BananaStock

A workout partner can boost your motivation by providing companionship and encouragement.

of any given class. Truly, the ladies from the 9:00 a.m. step class at Club X or the men and women at Club Z's Friday evening cycle class come to know each other by name, joke with each other, comment on improvements in each other, notice each other's absence, and ultimately motivate each other. In some fitness circles, societal interaction becomes so strong that participants both remember and celebrate each other's birthdays.

Group exercise participants seek out classes that make them feel comfortable. They may choose a similar spot in the room of any given group class, exercise with people whose fitness level most closely resembles their own, use a specific cycle, or attend only a specific instructor's classes, for example. Because of these dynamics, participants grow comfortable in the group exercise classes they choose. In such a relatively homogeneous environment, then, participants often meet, greet, and motivate each other. Indeed, some of the best group exercise classes occur when the difference between instructor and members is so small that everyone seems more like motivating friends than disconnected individuals in a room gathering to sweat to music.

Joining different types of groups can also help motivate you to work out with them. Your local YWCA, gyms, health clubs, and even spas sometimes offer groups dedicated to early morning cardio workouts, both indoors and outdoors. Furthermore, Internet providers now offer chat rooms and posting boards for a plethora of outdoor activities; simply visit, sign your name, and read the postings of where groups will gather for activities from running to dog walking. Cycling, rock climbing, running, hiking, and even aquatic groups meet regularly at these organizations. As always with Internet sites, always proceed with caution and common sense about venturing out to meet individuals or groups alone.

Groups motivate through the sheer number of people; more people create more energy and, as a consequence, the group dynamics create a supportive feeling of camaraderie. Another motivating factor of joining groups that specialize in outdoor activities is that, when weather conditions do not allow for going outdoors, the group may engage in a somewhat similar activity indoors, such as taking the outside cycling inside to attend a group cycling class. The activity remains engaging because, although you may have changed the venue, you have not changed the group!

No matter how you motivate yourself, remember that fitness is always both a journey and a destination. This will help you stay motivated by helping you enjoy each of your morning cardio workouts (your journey) while simultaneously keeping an eye on your goals (your destination).

2

Mind and Body Status Report

Perhaps you have thought about your fitness goals before this chapter. We are going to help you hone those goals via a complete, holistic approach to fitness that encompasses the brain, the body, and the breath. Furthermore, we will help you understand why this connection is so important so early in the day to set the tone for the entire day. We title this concept *carpe diem* because it signifies the early morning aspect of our book, the ability to "seize the day" early and maximize your body's potential as early as possible. In this chapter we will help you develop the connection between the mind and body as it pertains to your morning cardio workout. Understanding what we call the brain–body–breath connection is important in cardiovascular workouts because of the many aspects involved, from safety to motivation to intensity.

Your Internal Triangle

We believe that the body consists of three main parts: the brain, the body, and the breath. The body refers to our physiology: the conglomeration of muscles and bones that works for us in our morning cardio workouts. The brain refers to a concept of mindfulness, concentration, and awareness about our bodies moving through space and time during our chosen workouts. The breath refers to our ability to use our life force, what yogis call *prana*, to oxygenate our cells with the air around us. This breath is crucial to our workouts because, like food, it is a form of fuel. Taking a breath is the first thing you did when you came into this world, and regardless of how you leave the world, it will be the last thing you do. Therefore we emphasize the importance of the breath to maximize the efficacy of your morning cardio workouts. This emphasis of brain, body, and breath forms a thread throughout our book. Although the concept of brain–body–breath may at first appear daunting, we encourage you to be aware of it as you read this book. It may seem theoretical on the page, but you'll soon realize the interconnectedness of these elements in the workouts we propose for you in this book.

Keeping the brain–body–breath relationship in mind in the morning establishes a feeling of connectedness and centeredness in time and space. It also sets the tone for the rest of the day. Recent research shows that when exercisers concentrate on the quality of their movement and on their breath, they are more successful and have more endurance than when they are distracted about other things. The same

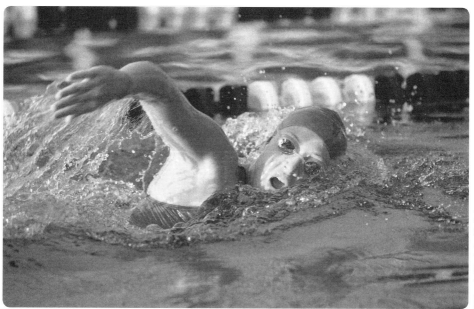

Breathing deeply and focusing on the quality of your movement will result in a more centered and rewarding workout.

sources say that when exercisers engage in such concentration early in the day, they are more likely to maintain that ability to concentrate during the rest of the day than if they engaged in such activities later in the day (American Council on Exercise 2004; Wilcox, Harford, and Wedel 1985). When you choose a morning cardio workout in a mindful way, you maximize the benefits of your goals, not only during that workout, but also for the rest of the day.

Learning to develop your own sense of interconnectedness among brain, body, and breath will help your workouts, and your life! Understanding this brain–body–breath connection will help you achieve a greater sense of yourself overall. This in turn will help you achieve additional goals as you set them because your self-discipline also will increase.

To develop this connection among brain, body, and breath, start your day by recognizing your feelings. Not everyone wakes up happy. Not everyone wakes up motivated to work out. Here's a suggestion for a way to stay abreast of your internal state. Table 2.1 is a log to use to record an ongoing list of the elements of your brain–body–breath connection. The purpose of such a log is twofold. First, having to translate the categories to numbers makes you analyze your feelings and become aware of them. Second, a log gives you a long-term record you can look back on to see trends and tendencies over time. For example, you may notice distinct differences between weekend days and workdays or between vacation and nonvacation days, or you may notice a lag during certain times of the month. If you notice that your motivation is always low during your monthly period or on workdays, for example, you can come up with strategies to boost your energy levels during those times, such as the motivation strategies discussed in chapter 1.

Before your morning cardio workout, choose a number between 1 and 10 for the items listed in the log, in which 1 signifies the lowest number and 10 signifies the highest number. Develop the discipline to fill out the log before and after every workout so that you can establish a trend and look back over your log after a week, a month, and perhaps longer. You will notice that we address objective items such as heart rate. The purpose is to help you note that, as your cardiovascular fitness increases, your heart rate should decrease. If it does not, consult your medical care practitioner. In addition to measuring quantifiable items such as heart rate, however, we include subjective items such as energy because examining both emotional and physical aspects helps you hone your awareness of the brain–body–breath connection.

When you take your resting heart rate later in the day after your workout (any time two hours after your workout), you must have been at rest (sitting or lying idle) for a minimum of one hour. When you take your morning heart rate, be sure you are in a quiet state. If you tend to jolt up because of an alarm, rest quietly for one minute before taking your pulse. Remember that the overall purpose of the log is to increase your awareness of your emotions regarding fitness and further develop the brain–body–breath connection. As you undertake more morning cardio workouts, you may want to make copies of the log so you have enough blank spaces to fill in.

Table 2.1 **Brain–Body–Breath Fitness Log**

Date _____

Workout chosen _____

Time invested in workout (warm-up to cool-down) _____

Resting heart rate: Upon wakening _____ After 1 hour of rest _____

	Before workout	After workout
BRAIN		
Stress level (1-10)		
Motivation level (1-10)		
Concentration level (high, medium, low)		
Adjectives (i.e., calm, anxious, focused, distracted)		
BODY		
Energy level (1-10)		
Adjectives (i.e., tense, achy, relaxed, energized, tired)		
BREATH		
Breathing quality (i.e., shallow, calm, deep, rhythmic, fast)		

Notes: _____
_____
_____
_____
_____
_____

From *Morning Cardio Workouts* by June E. Kahn and Lawrence J.M. Biscontini, 2007, Champaign, IL: Human Kinetics.

Setting Goals

Setting specific, attainable goals can help you achieve success. Imagine being out at sea on a sailboat. You see the horizon in the distance and set sail for it. The irony is that no matter how much distance you cover, you never get any closer. The horizon is unreachable. Likewise, putting your goals on the horizon is futile because you'll never attain them. For this reason, we suggest that you keep your goals close at hand by specifying and defining them often, not only to remind yourself of why you exercise, but also to make sure they are realistic. You may also want to show your goals to someone you trust. Fresh eyes can help you determine whether your goals are realistic. A fellow runner, personal trainer, or good friend may be able to give you valuable feedback on your goals.

Perhaps you work out simply because you enjoy it—whether it's the endorphin rush, the positive energy of a group workout, or even just the feeling of being reenergized, if you exercise because it brings you pleasure, pure enjoyment might be goal enough for you. Making a list of reasons and goals for your workouts will help you stay focused. This list may include improving your overall feelings, losing more body fat, feeling more energetic in the late afternoon, sleeping better, creating more endorphin rushes, and dropping a number in clothing size. When you write down your goals, try to be as specific as possible. For example, instead of saying "to improve my fitness level," you may say, "to lower my resting heart rate by a few beats." Make each goal specific and realistic.

When setting your goals, try to include those that address your brain, body, and breath. Our log gives you some examples. Your brain goals should refer to your concentration, thoughts, feelings, and sense of centeredness. Your body goals should be measurable goals that are objective and quantifiable with numbers. Finally, your breath goals should relate to the times you can become conscious of your breath, such as when working out, at rest, or when meditating.

Write your goals on a piece of paper, with "Carpe Diem" written boldly across the top. This title can help remind you of your commitment to capitalize on the day's potential early in the day. Pin your goals to the wall in a location that allows you to see and review them almost immediately upon awakening. As soon as you open your eyes in the morning, you will see your own self-created finish line. Having this list will help your motivation on those days when you find yourself dragging yourself out of bed for your cardio workouts. The title "Carpe Diem" will reiterate your commitment to *do it now*. If you work out with a personal trainer, you may want to share this list occasionally with him or her to help ascertain that your fitness goals are realistic. Furthermore, you will notice that the list is dated; you should update your goals as you evolve in many ways.

As you complete your goal list, consider the following questions:

- Does at least one goal address the brain (i.e., your mental outlook, emotions, and feelings)? An example of a brain goal is "To feel more alert in the morning."

- Does at least one goal address the body (i.e., clothing sizes, measurable distances, or specific intensity numbers)? An example of a body goal is "To lower my resting heart rate."
- Does at least one goal address the breath and spirit (i.e., your capacity to process air, to work harder, to increase intensity without being winded or breathless, to be able to take deeper breaths at will, such as when you are feeling stressed)? An example of a breath goal is "To take deeper breaths when feeling stressed."

Perhaps the most exciting outcome of the morning cardio workout programs we've created for you will be the release of endorphins. As we mentioned earlier, these chemicals, which are released among the neurotransmitters of the brain, help you stay consistent in fitness because they make you feel energized, happy, and even excited. Many of our long-term fitness goals (such as fat loss) take a while to realize; endorphins, however, serve as immediate gratification during and after the workout.

Mental Preparation

As we discussed earlier, mental concentration plays an important role in the brain–body–breath connection. Socrates in ancient Greece said that "the unexamined life is not worth living," which demonstrates the point that keeping a constant awareness of our feelings is important. Another Greek philosophical proverb, equally old, rephrases our carpe diem theme nicely: "If it's worth doing, the only time to do it is early in the morning." In modern-day Greece, this has evolved into the following ubiquitous motto: "Early, early, do it with the dawn!"

In our book we capitalize on this ancient concept of maximizing your abilities as early in the day as possible to take advantage of yourself when you are the freshest. Begin the day developing your sense of who you are as you align your brain, body, and breath. An awareness of your mental outlook is key. Furthermore, because each day is a fresh start, we remind you to make every effort to live in the present and make each workout and each day count. The following adage may help you understand the value of each day:

> Yesterday is history;
> Tomorrow is a mystery.
> Today is a special gift;
> That's why we call it *the present.*

Records from the ancient Greeks, Romans, and Turks in the first gymnasiums show that physical exercise was done in the morning, and the term *carpe diem* developed as a result. "Grabbing the day" originally meant grabbing the day for physical exertion, and each day was seen as a new opportunity to do just that

(Hamilton 1998). Instead of focusing on the past or future, remember that the current workout is the only one that matters.

Sometimes we can be so aware of our brain–body–breath connection that we can be overly judgmental of ourselves. If we miss a workout or work out at an intensity that is less than our goal, we may feel guilty. Guilt can prevent us from achieving our best in the present moment. It may help you to remember that guilt is a negative emotion that can only be associated with the past (you can't be guilty of the present or future). Because we are focusing on the present as we seek to develop our carpe diem brain–body–breath connection, we shouldn't have guilt as an emotion in our fitness endeavors.

In discussing carpe diem, the subject of time management arises and just *when* is the ideal time to seize the day. Among the most useful suggestions we can give you is to budget, plan, and schedule the time you need for your morning cardio workout. If you have a daily scheduling tool for blocking out time, such as a PDA (personal digital assistant), block out specific times for morning cardio workouts. If you do, you will be more likely to be diligent and punctual about your workout in the same way you would for a doctor, dentist, travel, or work appointment. Be sure to specify, if only briefly, some of your brain–body–breath goals. For example, your entry may read like this:

5:15 a.m. Body: Treadmill/bike routine
           Brain: Concentrate on endurance
           Breath: Work at intensity for mouth breathing

Or

6:30 a.m. Body: 30-minute outdoor run
           Brain: Concentrate on footfall form
           Breath: Awareness of outdoor scents

In the evening, as you review your schedule for the following day, you will see your morning cardio workout scheduled with priority at the start of the day. This will help you prepare mentally and reinforce your dedication to an attitude of carpe diem for the following day. Having that dedicated time in your schedule for your morning cardio workout can help reinforce the brain–body–breath connection because you are reaffirming your commitment to your goals first thing the following morning. In addition, the more you refer to your brain–body–breath goals for the following day, the more they will remain in the forefront of your mind instead of cropping up unexpectedly the next day.

In conclusion, remember that your morning cardio workouts are not just designed to train the body. Once you are aware of the brain–body–breath connection, you will notice the improvements as you train each of these systems. Keeping a journal in which you record your feelings and stress levels, for example, will help you track your progress over time in addition to tracking merely whether you accomplished your workouts. Keeping an objective, measurable list of your goals where you can see them before your morning workouts will help you stay focused on your goals. Finally, enjoying the endorphins in the brain will help you appreciate the brain–body–breath connection as you reach your goals.

3

Muscles in Motion

When you engage in your morning cardio workout, it's easy to lose sight of all of the muscles and organs that work together for you in your brain–body–breath connection. Even if you read this chapter only once, it will help you understand how the muscles of both the upper and lower body connect through the core, even when you are not consciously aware of them during a run, for example. So many aspects of the body fuse for the purpose of helping you achieve your goals. Because your workout takes place so early as you seize the day, it's easy to enjoy the workout without thinking of the many aspects of the body that come together as you work out. Let's take a moment to look at the muscles independently—including the heart itself—and then look at how they work together to get you warmed up for your brain–body–breath workout. Being aware of how the muscles in your body come together will enhance your brain–body–breath connection and help you achieve your early morning cardio workout goals.

Anatomy of a Cardio Workout

Because the body is part of our brain–body–breath trilogy, spending a bit of time understanding how your body works for you like a fine-tuned machine will give you a deeper appreciation for your workout. The purpose of this section is to give you an understanding of the major muscles involved in producing the power you need for your morning cardio workouts. To be sure, all of the workouts described in this book will maximize the benefits to your heart, but other muscles are crucial as well. We will look at muscles in both the upper and lower body that produce the power you need, the tendons and ligaments that hold it all together, and the all-important heart.

The purpose of discussing upper- and lower-body muscles is to increase your overall awareness of the muscles that help your heart achieve its cardiovascular goals of getting stronger, improving $\dot{V}O_2$max, becoming more efficient to pump more blood with each contraction, and lowering its resting heart rate. Even though each muscle has its clearly defined and unique function, all the muscles in the body come together for this main cardiovascular goal. Injury occurs when we neglect or improperly warm up a certain body part. Sometimes imbalances occur. Our strategy, then, is to understand how the muscles work and help them warm up in the most efficient way possible.

Muscles

Muscles are groups of tissues that cross joints in the body. When they contract, they produce movement by shortening the distance between the joints. When your biceps muscles—which run down your arms and cross your elbows—contract, your elbow bends (flexes). Similarly, all movement in your body takes place when the distance between your joints shortens. Because muscles contract and expand at extremely fast rates thousands of times during your morning cardio workout, both proper warm-up and stretching of these muscles are important to promote efficient movement and prevent injury. The muscles of the calf, for example, will contract thousands of times during a run. If you finish a run without stretching those muscles, they can stay contracted, leading to injury.

The specific major muscles used during your morning cardio workouts appear in figures 3.1 and 3.2. The names may seem complicated, but they are recognized internationally because we still refer to them by their original Latin and Greek names. The purpose of providing these figures is to give you a better understanding of where muscles are located in your body and what their names are. Some people find it interesting to learn that the muscles we commonly refer to as "chest muscles" actually are called the pectoralis major group. If you can identify the muscles involved in your routine by name, such as "gastrocnemius" for the calf muscle used during an uphill treadmill walk, your brain–body–breath awareness is that much greater. You can then concentrate on the contractions of those muscles with every conscious, mindful footfall. Repeating to yourself such things as, "my gastrocnemii are working, so my heart benefits," or "I feel my gastrocnemius contract every time my heel strikes the treadmill," are examples of using this information to increase your body awareness.

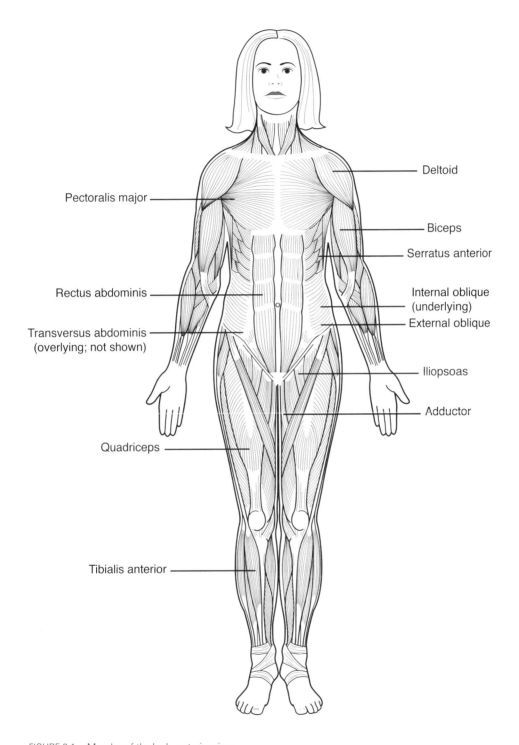

Deltoid

Pectoralis major

Biceps

Serratus anterior

Rectus abdominis

Internal oblique
(underlying)

External oblique

Transversus abdominis
(overlying; not shown)

Iliopsoas

Adductor

Quadriceps

Tibialis anterior

FIGURE 3.1   Muscles of the body, anterior view.

Reprinted, by permission, from S. Cole, 2003, *Athletic abs* (Champaign, IL: Human Kinetics), 24.

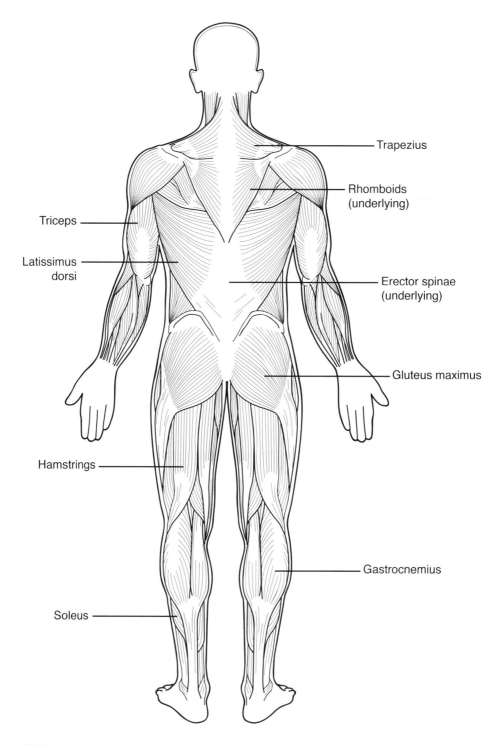

FIGURE 3.2   Muscles of the body, posterior view.

Reprinted, by permission, from S. Cole, 2003, *Athletic abs* (Champaign, IL: Human Kinetics), 24.

Lower-Body Muscles Many of the morning cardio workouts we provide in this book involve supporting your own body weight on the muscles of the lower extremities. To be sure, not all workouts involve working all muscles evenly, so an awareness of what muscles you are using in any particular workout will help you balance other muscles in subsequent workouts to avoid imbalance. Muscular imbalance—using the same muscles over and over so that some get stronger and some get weaker—can lead to injury. Whenever you engage in a modality that involves your own support of your body weight (which is almost any activity except sitting on a bike or using a rowing machine), you involve the muscles of the lower legs that work together: the anterior tibialis (shin) and gastrocnemius/soleus (calf) group. Because most cardiovascular exercise (e.g., walking, running, stepping) involves pushing the foot downward as you move forward, the anterior muscles (along the front of the lower leg) often get neglected, which can lead to muscular imbalance. Certain exercises can help diminish this imbalance. Doing just three sets of 12 repetitions of toe raises when you are not involved in your morning cardio workout can diminish this imbalance and increase your overall safety.

Moving up the leg, we find the muscles that run down the back of the upper leg, collectively called the hamstring group. These flex (bend) the knee and extend the hip, which means they help take your leg behind your body. Down the front of the upper leg are the quadriceps, which extend (straighten) the knee and flex (bend) the hip, such as when you are running forward or stepping up and down from a platform. Working both of these opposing muscle groups is important to avoid muscle overuse and imbalance. A good way to do this is to combine some step training with running, walking, or jogging.

Upper-Body Muscles Although you may think that the muscles of the upper body are involved very little in your cardiovascular routines, a closer study will reveal that they play a significant role. The muscles of the chest, the pectoralis major, help support the body when upright, help move the arms, and assist in posture. Their opposing muscles on the back that form a trapezoid, the trapezius, help with similar functions. We are a forward-oriented society. We hunch and round our spine in almost all of our activities: preparing food, sitting and eating, reading, sitting at a work desk and checking e-mail, driving, and even sleeping for hours on end in a curled position. Incorporating our trapezius muscles into our routines will help prevent imbalances and improve overall posture. Working the trapezius improves posture by pulling the shoulders back and correcting the imbalance of a stronger pectoralis muscle. Doing just three sets of 12 repetitions of shoulder squeezes behind you when seated can help your overall safety and diminish imbalances of the upper body. To perform a shoulder squeeze, imagine that someone has just poured a pitcher of ice-cold water down your back; you react to the cold water by sitting erect and squeezing your shoulder blades together behind you. Repeat this for three sets of 12 repetitions.

The muscles of the shoulders, the deltoids, move your arms in all directions during your cardiovascular workouts, whether you are performing complex arm choreography in a group exercise class or simply moving your arms forward and backward during a run. The muscles in the front of the arm that bend the elbow (the biceps) and the muscles down the back of the upper arm that bend the elbow against resistance (the triceps) assist in everyday activities, as well as morning cardio workouts. Natural arm movements occur when we are standing, walking, running, cycling, or stepping. During group exercise, new arm movement patterns are created. An awareness of the muscles in the arms (that both bend and straighten the elbow) can help minimize muscular imbalances. Usually the deltoids in the front of the shoulder are stronger than those in the back, so repeating the same shoulder squeezes as described for strengthening the trapezius, this time with your elbows out to the sides and parallel to the floor, can help your overall safety and diminish imbalances.

Core Muscles The nucleus, or core, of the body can be described as anything that attaches to the spinal column or crosses the shoulders or hips. Many people direct their attention immediately to the muscles that run vertically in front of their torso (rectus abdominis) when initially asked to touch their core. However, it's important to realize that the core encompasses the muscles to the sides of the torso that help you twist (the obliques), the muscles that run vertically up the back that help you sit upright and bend backward (the spinal erectors), the deep pelvic floor muscles that control elimination and sexual function, and the ever-so-important muscles around the midsection that help draw in the waistline to give active, internal support at all times (the transverse abdominis). Being able to draw your navel in toward your spine during all activities, especially your morning cardio workouts, is crucial to working the core because this helps you find stability and prevents all types of injuries (Cook 1998).

The more you can maintain the spine in a safe, neutral position, the more you can do to diminish the chances of injury. To achieve a neutral spine, all of the aforementioned muscles work together to keep you safe. The rectus abdominis between the ribs and the hips helps pull you forward, such as when you bend over to pick something up. The spinal erectors running down your spine help pull you backward, such as when you bend back in the shower to shampoo your hair. The obliques located on either side of your core help rotate you to each side, such as when you sit in a car and twist to one side to get the seatbelt and then twist to the other to fasten it. When all of these muscles work together, called "synergism," they each pull on the spine in such a way that the spine remains tall. There is equal static tension from all of these muscles, and the core remains neutral. During exercise, the more we can maintain this static tension of these core muscles, the safer we will remain. If we consistently train one of the core muscles more than the others, muscular imbalances may result. For example, if we always do abdominal curls (flexions) and never work the spinal extensors (extension), we could end up with a rounded (forward flexed) posture due to this muscular imbalance.

Most intimately, the core consists of the muscles that comprise the pelvic floor. These are the muscles that control elimination functions. If you have had children and practiced Kegel exercises during childbirth preparation, you practiced working out your pelvic floor muscles. These are the most internal muscles of your core, and you can and should train them with regularity. Training the muscles of the pelvic floor is easy, and men should do these exercises also. Become aware of the muscles that control the bodily functions of elimination of both solid and liquid. Try to squeeze and close these muscles, then release. Repeat this at least 12 times. During your morning cardio workouts it's important to maintain a strong pelvic floor by keeping it slightly contracted. This will increase stability and support as you add mobility, prevent incontinence, increase overall control, and train the body from the inside out as you move. (Chek 2004). The more you strengthen the pelvic muscles, the more naturally it will feel to contract them during your morning cardio workout. Keeping the pelvic floor partially contracted also strengthens the brain–body–breath connection because it takes mental power (brain) to engage those deep pelvic muscles during another activity such as a run (body), while being conscious of your breathing the entire time (breath).

Ligaments and Tendons

In addition to understanding muscles, it's important to understand the structures that connect muscles to bones (tendons) and bones to bones (ligaments). Proper warm-ups will keep these structures strong and injury free. Ligaments connect bone to bone and do get stronger with cardiovascular exercise. They are not designed to stretch but to support the skeletal system and help it move. Many important ligaments are found in the ankles, for example, and help the bones of the ankle move in a wide variety of ways. Injuries often occur in ligaments when they stretch and the connecting bones hyperextend, or lock. For example, if you stand tall so your legs are straight and try to straighten even more, pushing the backs of the knees behind you, this action (called hyperextension) could result in the stretching of the medial knee ligaments. Because these ligaments are not supposed to stretch, injury could result from improper posture and a locking out of the knees during exercise.

To avoid stretching a ligament or hyperextending joints (locking open an elbow or knee), you need a proper warm-up, which means (1) a gradual increase in temperature around the muscles and ligaments, (2) a rhythmic rehearsal that is specific to the activity, and (3) some type of stretching of the area to be worked. Furthermore, a strong attention to alignment during all phases of your morning cardio workouts and a proper flexibility routine (appropriate stretching of used muscles from 10 to 30 seconds at least three times per week) following your workout will help decrease injury.

Tendons connect muscle to bone and also get stronger with cardiovascular exercise. They are designed to be flexible, but not to increase measurably in length over time during or after exercise. They are like strong, thick rubber bands that can stretch slightly but prefer to remain at a constant length. An example of an important tendon is the one behind the lower leg referred to as the Achilles tendon. It connects the gastrocnemius calf muscle to the calcaneous, or heel. To keep tendons healthy, the same guidelines for a proper warm-up offered in the proceeding paragraph apply.

Heart

We turn now to a "heart-to-heart" chat about the reason you picked up this book. The heart is a skeletal muscle located in the center of your chest that serves as your nonstop pump. From the time you leave your mother's womb until you leave the world, it will not stop. The heart has four chambers, as seen in figure 3.3. Blood from all over the body gets "tired" and deoxygenated and needs a freshening up from the lungs. It enters the heart through the venae cavae into the right atrium cavity, continues through the lower-right ventricle cavity, and then travels to the lungs where capillaries give it fresh oxygen. From the lungs, this blood returns to the heart via the pulmonary veins, entering through the upper-left atrium cavity. It passes through the lower-left ventricle cavity, and then gets pumped via the aorta throughout the body and to the muscles where it is used for exercise and other activities. When you look at the figure 3.3, you will notice that the traditional sides of left and right are reversed. This is because the heart diagram depicts the actual position of chambers in the heart as the heart appears inside the human body. If you hold this page up to your body and turn it around to face away from you, then the diagram depicts the right and left sides of the heart correctly.

During your cardiovascular workout, the blood-pumping system accelerates. Blood pressure and heart rate increase as the heart pumps a greater volume of blood than it does when you are at rest. As a result of chemical reactions in the body during the aerobic system of processing more oxygen, more waste products are produced, which are carbon dioxide (you exhale more) and water (you sweat more). As intensity decreases, both blood pressure and heart rate decrease. In this section we discuss heart rate and blood pressure in more detail.

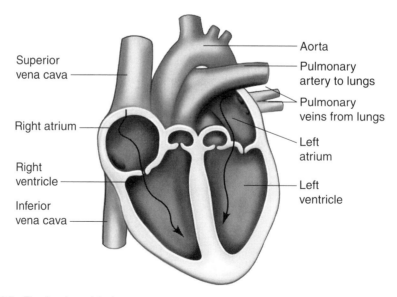

FIGURE 3.3   The chambers of the heart.

Reprinted, by permission, from B. Sharkey, 2002, *Fitness and health*, 5th ed. (Champaign, IL: Human Kinetics), 91.

Heart Rate If you want to monitor your heart's improvement over time as a result of your morning cardio workouts, you should learn about heart rate training. The purpose of heart rate training is to be able to gauge with more precision your heart's intensity. In chapter 2 we encouraged you to record your resting heart rate so you notice over time whether it decreases as your heart's efficiency increases. During a workout, you can find a specific zone in which to work by using an industry-accepted formula for determining your target heart rate range. Because you will become more aware (brain) of your heart rate over time at different stages of your workouts (body), you may also consider purchasing a heart rate monitor. This device enables you to determine instantly your heart rate during a workout with much more ease than trying to maintain a given intensity and count your pulse manually.

To determine your target heart rate range, use this simplified formula:

(220 – your age) × % of intensity range (65 to 90%)

For example, if you are 45 years old, 220 – 45 = 175. Therefore, 175 is your maximum heart rate. You usually will not work out at your maximum heart rate, but rather between 65 percent (the low end) and 90 percent (the upper end) of your maximum heart rate. To calculate the beats per minute for these ranges, use the following formulas:

175 × .65 (the low end of your range) = 114 beats per minute

175 × .90 (the upper end of your range) = 158 beats per minute

You should try to achieve a heart rate between 114 and 158 beats per minute for most of your morning cardio workout. To *maintain* your fitness level, you should stay closer to the lower end; to *improve* your fitness level, you should work at an intensity that allows your heart rate to remain around 158 beats per minute. Another way to explain this is to say that the newer you are to working out, the closer you will want to stay to the low end of your hart rate range. The more you want to challenge yourself, the higher you should work in your range. We suggest you take your heart rate after your initial five minutes, and then monitor it at least twice during the bulk of your workout. At the end of your workout, be sure that your heart rate has come down out of that range. If not, walking for a few minutes may help your rate return to a more normal state. You will be keenly aware of your brain–body–breath connection as you learn to work out between the upper and lower end of your heart rate range.

Consciously making the heart work harder and then giving it ample time to rest trains it to respond faster and more efficiently to everyday tasks that are not as consciously focused on the heart. Your morning cardio workouts will give you all of the benefits we have been discussing, but most importantly, they will train your heart to become stronger. The heart of an average untrained adult beats between 70 and 80 times per minute at rest. You will notice that the workouts in this book will help you decrease that number. The reason is that, as your heart becomes more efficient, it pumps more blood with each contraction, necessitating fewer pumps per minute. Over time, then, your resting heart rate should decrease if you are not on caffeine or medication that can interfere with this process. The benefits of a lower resting heart rate include a more efficient heart, a stronger circulatory system, and a more efficient cardiopulmonary system.

Blood Pressure   In one minute your heart pumps about five liters of blood. When your heart contracts and relaxes, this massaging action pushes the blood through the heart to its appropriate destination. When the heart contracts, a certain amount of pressure is created. This contraction is called the systole, and its number results in a systolic reading. Similarly, when the heart relaxes, the resulting pressure is called the diastole, whose number results in a diastolic reading.

The traditional medical recommendation for normal blood pressure readings at rest is 120/80 mmHg (American College of Sports Medicine 1998). When blood pressure gets higher, the body becomes at risk for cardiopulmonary issues such as heart attacks and strokes because the system isn't working as efficiently as it could be. The good news is that morning cardio workouts can help lower blood pressure without medication. An awareness of your resting blood pressure can give you an indication of your general health and also enhance your brain–body–breath connection

Injury Prevention

The purpose of this section is to review the components of a workout that should come together to make your workout the safest possible experience. Although there are many factors you cannot control, such as traffic and weather, going over a checklist of the things you can control will help you move safely toward your goals. To prevent injury, the acronym BALANCE is key.

- **B = Balance in everything.** Choose morning cardio workouts that balance each other in intensity. Balance interval workouts with steady state training. Balance longer workout times with shorter times. Balance full weight-bearing training with some non-weight-bearing training such as seated machines and aquatics. Balance workouts that use specialized equipment with workouts that rely on no equipment except your brain, body, and breath. Balance workouts that primarily address the muscles down the front of the leg with those that address the muscles down the back of the leg. Also, build flexibility into your morning cardio workouts, both before (to help the muscles prepare) and after (to help the muscles recover).

- **A = Always choose your workouts based on realistic goals.** When choosing a morning cardio workout, be sure to read the purpose of the workout so you understand whether this will serve as a building block toward your overall goals. If your goal is to lose a pound of body fat per week, then choosing some workouts that extend beyond 20 minutes and that offer intervals can help you reach your goal. If, however, your goal is to maintain where you are in terms of body fat, interval programs may not be for you because they can result in a reduction in overall mass because of their intensity. Remember that you must also choose the appropriate movements for the warm-up phase of the workout to help prevent injury.

Two other factors to consider in your selection are your overall enjoyment and your uniqueness. Choose an activity that you know you will enjoy and that your body will respond to with a healthier brain–body–breath union rather than one you will dread from the moment you awaken. Also, respect your uniqueness. If you do not enjoy taking long interval runs outside alone, but enjoy the dynamics of a group, then seek out different types of classes that meet your needs.

- **L = Ligaments, tendons, and muscles.** Make sure the start and end of your workout addresses ligaments, tendons, and muscles. Remember to increase gradually both your body temperature and the range of motion of these structures to reduce the risk of injury. Paying attention to flexibility before and after your morning cardio workout will help decrease the potential for injury. In developing and training your brain–body–breath connection, taking a moment now and then to think about your ligaments, tendons, and muscles and how they work synergistically toward your goals can help increase your overall self-awareness and mindfulness. This process will help you achieve more success in your workout because concentrating on different body parts can involve them more efficiently.

- **A = Align your body with your brain and breath.** This reiterates our mission of involving the brain, body, and breath in your workouts. You may find that exercising early in the morning carries with it the temptation to partially wake up, put on your shoes in a sleepy state, and start moving without a conscious realization of the task at hand. Taking just a minute to review your goals, fill in the questions from your pre- and postworkout chart in chapter 2, review your carpe diem list from chapter 2, and take a full breath will help align your brain, body, and breath for your workout. Neglecting to do so could mean the potential for injury because your body may not be fully awake and realize the work that is about to ensue. Mindfulness is all!

- **N = Need for rest and recovery.** Before embarking on any morning cardio workout, be sure to listen to your body's messages. Do you have pain? Are you sore? Does something feel tight? Working through pain is a sure way to increase the likelihood for injury. Most important, use your brain–body–breath awareness to focus on your feelings about your body. Be sure you feel adequately rested before engaging in an intense workout. If you do not, vary your intensity accordingly. Avoid working through pain or soreness. Working through existing pain may hurt you more than help you. Being sore before your workout may mean that you have been ignoring an integral part of any morning cardio workout, the recovery phase. Proper amounts of sleep form part of this rest and recovery protocol. Remember that you need to rest and recover as intensively as you train.

- **C = Check your shoes, your apparel, and the weather.** This point will help you avoid injury by being the most prepared, from your feet to your head. Shoe selection should be appropriate to the task at hand. Your apparel should promote your skin's ability to breathe, dissipate heat, and sweat easily. From choosing shoes that are designed for the terrain you will encounter to selecting apparel that will protect you from the rain, taking a moment for this point in our checklist will help keep you safe, dry, and injury free.

• **E = Educate yourself about your body.** Balance comes from an alignment and awareness of the brain–body–breath connection. Learn to be in touch with your feelings about stress, energy, and emotions. Learn to identify different types of morning cardio workouts to help you change the stimuli so that your body can react to different types of fitness protocols. This book gives you a plethora of examples. During your workouts, you are taxing the heart and other systems beyond their normal capacity at rest. You may wonder, How should this workout or exercise feel? During a workout, you should feel as though you are working, including experiencing a mild discomfort that is *not* painful. During cardiovascular exercise, you should feel winded but not breathless. Being able to speak in short sentences is a good gauge of whether your intensity is too high; as long as you can manage to speak, then you most probably are working at an appropriate intensity. Not being able to breathe or answer questions with ease during exercise means you need to lower your intensity. Learning how to recognize the differences between discomfort and pain can take time. Pain is sharp, often quick, and throbbing. Pain is the body's message that you the need to seek medical attention for proper diagnosis and appropriate treatment. Educate yourself about the best intensity for you given your realistic goals.

In part two you will learn about preferred intensity and perceived exertion. Your workout goal for a given morning, as well as how you feel, will determine the intensity at which to work. Even during a steady state, light workout you will want to work at an intensity that will allow you to be aware of your breath and body responses.

After a workout, you may experience delayed onset muscle soreness, often referred to as DOMS, for short. This is a feeling of soreness in a specific muscular area or areas experienced between 24 and 48 hours after exercising. It comes from the tiny muscular tears that happen when you tax the muscular system beyond its normal capacity, or when you use muscles in a different muscular pattern for the first time. If you try a new cardiovascular machine for the first time, or attend a new group fitness class, you may find soreness in specific areas on the following day because the body is not accustomed to the new patterns of movement; in a way, your body was shocked into learning. If you continue to use the same machine or attend the same class, however, your muscles will adapt and the feelings of soreness will decrease. Your morning cardio workouts will change the way your body moves, and some workouts may make you more sore than others will. You will learn that the soreness produced from mild discomfort is your body's message that you've accomplished work in moving toward your fitness goals. Remember that soreness that occurs as a result of new cardiovascular workouts is never a long-lasting experience.

Warming Up

Now that you know the basics of how the body works in cardiovascular exercise and are aware of how to prevent injuries, it's time to start warming up for your brain–body–breath morning cardio workout. As you prepare for the plethora of options of workouts offered in this book, remember that some type of warm-up is necessary to reduce the risk of injury; allow the muscles, tendons, and ligaments discussed earlier in this chapter to work efficiently; raise the body's intensity gradually; and create an overall more productive workout experience.

A warm-up can consist of many different types of movements. No one specific warm-up is appropriate for everyone, or for every activity, for that matter. What is important is to engage the entire body in movements that make you warmer, either almost to the point of sweating or breaking a light sweat. Also, a warm-up should be somewhat specific to the activity you will do so the specific muscles will benefit. Doing biceps curls with light weights as a warm-up before a run may indeed warm you up, but the warm-up does nothing *specific* to the leg muscles you will use during the run. Examples of full-body warm-ups are walking, tai chi, running at a low intensity, or a combination of full arm circles and squats.

Perhaps the most important goal of a warm-up is a gradual rise in corporal temperature. The muscles, tendons, ligaments, and even organs need to experience a gradual rise in temperature before reaching their steady state of cardiovascular maintenance. For example, warming up only the legs before a run pays attention only to the lower body instead of providing some thermal benefits to the shoulders and arms, whose muscles also are involved quite critically in the run itself. If the entire body isn't warm before the activity, it may be too stiff to respond appropriately as the body increases intensity. Consequently, it may be prone to injury. When your entire body has increased its temperature before beginning the workout, your workout will be more effective in terms of maximizing benefits and diminishing risks (American Council on Exercise 2003; Gladwin 2003).

Safety first means a gradual increase in intensity. Shocking the body from its state of morning sleep into a sudden explosion of taxation can prove dangerous for both the circulatory and muscular systems. Instead, a gradual increase in intensity will help your body's many systems wake up and begin to work for you. A slow warm-up helps tell the muscles to prepare, not only for the activities of daily life, but also for the more intense workout experience about to ensue. In the following sections we discuss the two types of stretching and also provide some sample warm-up activities.

Stretching

Stretching specifics for the warm-up continue to be a controversy in the fitness and sport industries. Some experts have proven that static stretching before a cardiovascular activity decreases injury, and other experts have proven that stretching before an activity does nothing to diminish injury. Still other experts have proven that, in uniquely intense sport activities such as Olympic activities, preactivity stretching decreases strength and overall performance. For the purposes of this book and safety in your morning cardio workouts, we recommend that every warm-up include a combination of two types of stretching: active and static.

- **Active stretching.** Active stretching (sometimes called dynamic stretching) means working a muscle slowly and rhythmically to stretch its opposing muscle. Rhythmically stretching a muscle helps limber it as it warms up, making the muscle less prone to injury. An example of dynamic stretching is sitting on the edge of a chair and extending your knees so your heels face away from you. In this stretch you are working the quadriceps muscles that run down the front of your thighs, using them to extend your legs. More important to our task at hand, you are stretching the muscles down the back of the thigh called the hamstrings. You can do a series of 10 slowly, straightening the knees to a count of 5 and lowering the feet back to the floor for a count of 5. This will increase the temperature and mobility of the hamstring muscles as they prepare for work during the morning cardio workout.

- **Static stretching.** Static stretching means holding a muscle's stretch as you isolate that muscle, often using the floor, a stretching strap, or a wall. To stretch the hamstrings in a passive stretch, you can sit again on the edge of your chair and put the heels of your feet on the floor far enough away from you so that your knees are not flexed (bent). With your upper body extended and lengthened, bend forward from your hips (not your waist) without rounding your spine until you feel a stretch down the backs of your legs. Hold this passive stretch for 10 to 30 seconds, and repeat twice.

Based on our experiences as personal trainers of consumers and athletes, and as group exercise instructors, we have seen injuries occur only in people who have engaged in activities without stretching first. We recommend active stretching in the warm-up because the goal is to warm up and rehearse the muscles. We recommend passive stretching after the cardiovascular workout because flexibility gains come from static stretching, and this is the goal of the postcardio stretch. Both of these types of stretching techniques will limber up your body prior to your morning cardio workouts and help you prevent injury. Following are a couple of stretches we recommend.

- **Chest stretch.** For a great stretch to the chest muscles, sit or stand and open your arms out to the sides as if preparing to give a big hug. Concentrate on the chest muscles about to be stretched. Instead of hugging someone, inhale and simultaneously move your arms farther behind you, as if preparing for an even bigger hug (see figure 3.4). Hold this for a minimum of 20 seconds, maintaining an awareness of your breath and body.

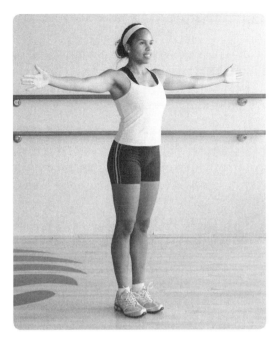

FIGURE 3.4   Chest stretch.

• **Gluteal muscle stretch.** For a great stretch for the gluteal muscles involved so much in cardio workouts involving the legs, sit upright and cross one ankle over the opposite knee. Concentrate on the deep gluteal muscles about to be stretched. As you breathe, slowly lower the knee of the lifted leg in the direction of the floor until you feel a deep stretch in the gluteal area (see figure 3.5). Hold this for a minimum of 20 seconds, maintaining an awareness of your breath and body.

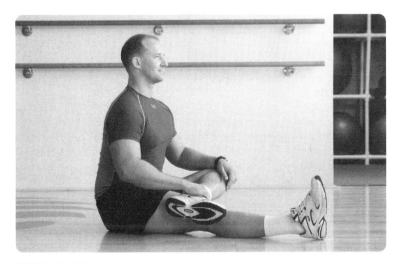

FIGURE 3.5   Gluteal muscle stretch.

Sample Warm-Up Activities

In addition to active and passive stretching, remember that your warm-up must be specific to your morning cardio workouts. If you are planning some type of weight-bearing outdoor activity such as a run, a walk, or an interval format, you need to pay attention to the muscles of your lower legs, spine, and the shoulders and arms. For example, to get ready for a morning walk or run, begin with a light to moderate walk for about three to five minutes, then take a few moments to warm up the low back by descending to a squat position and do the cat stretch. Flexing forward and placing your hands on your thighs, round your spine into a catlike position and hold for a few seconds (see figure 3.6a). Return to your neutral posture and then open up your chest and extend your spine, allowing your tailbone to point back and up (see figure 3.6b).

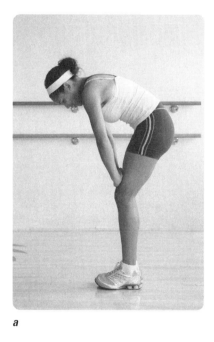
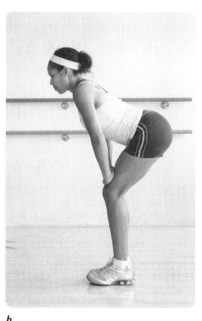

a   b

FIGURE 3.6   Cat stretch.

Repeat this walking and stretching process a few times back and forth and then continue to walk, increasing the pace to increase the intensity for a few minutes, and then stop to mildly stretch the hamstrings, calves, and quadriceps. Here are some stretches that will help you do just that:

• **Standing static one-leg hip hinge.** Stand with one foot forward and one foot back. Straighten your front leg and bend your back knee. Lean forward, pivoting at the hips, and place your hands on the thigh of your bent knee (see figure 3.7). Hold for 10 to 30 seconds. Repeat with your other leg.

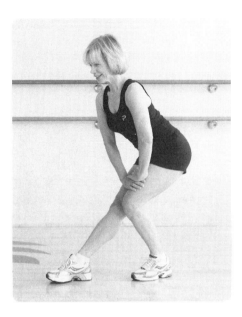

FIGURE 3.7   Standing static one-leg hip hinge.

• **Standing quadriceps static knee bend.** Stand with your feet together. Bend one knee and hold your ankle with the same-side hand; pull the heel toward the gluteals (see figure 3.8). Hold the stretch for 10 to 30 seconds. Repeat with your other leg. Touch a wall or hold onto something for balance if necessary.

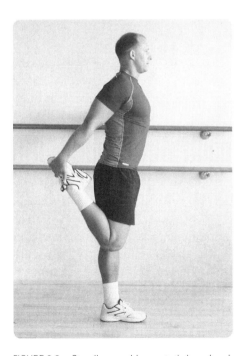

FIGURE 3.8   Standing quadriceps static knee bend.

- **Calf static heel press.** Stand with one foot forward and one foot back and your legs hip-width apart, feet facing forward. Bend your front knee and place your hands on your front thigh (see figure 3.9). Hold the stretch for 10 to 30 seconds. Repeat with your other leg.

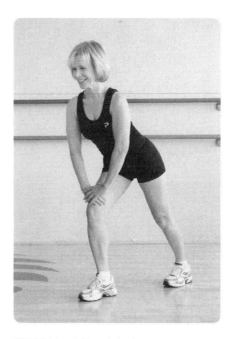

FIGURE 3.9   Calf static heel press.

A fundamental body part that often is forgotten before any type of morning cardio workout is the low back. The Aerobics and Fitness Association of America states that 80 percent of North Americans complain of low back pain (Gladwin 2003). Because the low back is where so many of the core muscles both connect and pass through, this area needs proper attention in the warm-up, during exercise, and after your workout. Because of the five large vertebrae of the lower spine here, plus the musculature of the area, it can be a particularly vulnerable part of the body if proper body mechanics are not observed. To stretch the low back in a biomechanically advantageous position, sit on the edge of a chair or a stability ball. Place your hands on your knees and round (forward flex) your back, concentrating on stretching your entire spine forward mindfully, from your neck to your low back area. It's not a lean forward; it's a rounding of each vertebra of the spine. Think of your spine as a column of very small, round doughnuts. Lean forward in such as way that you bring each doughnut forward separately. Maintain a mindful breath throughout. For a deeper stretch, continue breathing as you let your hands slide down your legs toward your ankles. Relax any tension in your shoulders. Be sure to continue touching your ankles, shoes, or the floor to avoid just dangling without support because this puts a dangerous stretch on the longitudinal ligament that runs down the spine.

Although there is no ideal warm-up for every person and every type of morning cardio workout, the following premise will help summarize your goals during this important phase of your workout: A warm-up should provide a gradual increase in intensity while allowing the body to increase its range of motion and engage in rhythmic, limbering movements that are specific to the activity about to be performed.

4

Outdoor Activities

‖‖

Do you enjoy the early morning sunshine, cool wind on your face, the changing of the seasons? Outdoor workouts allow you to get some fresh air and a change of scenery while giving you the opportunity to challenge your body against the elements of nature. Working against wind as well as other elements can certainly add to the variety of challenges to your system and often adds to the intensity of the workout, creating significant opportunities for your body to adapt and adjust to these changes. Whereas indoor exercises such as stationary biking and treadmill running (discussed in chapter 5) will certainly help you achieve your goals, taking your workout outdoors will add a new dimension to your fitness plan. Outdoor workouts offer a change in your workout plan every time because you must make automatic adjustments to changing weather conditions.

This chapter is designed to give you useful information as we explore the many popular options available for taking your morning workouts outside. For each activity listed, we review the common physical actions and the major muscles worked as well as proper form and technique. In addition, we offer tips on how to choose the equipment for the activity as well as safety tips to help you get the most out of your workout.

Walking

Walking is a popular, accessible, low-cost activity that can be done at a variety of intensities. People at all fitness levels can do walking workouts, and research indicates that the health benefits are many. Walking at a moderate to brisk pace can enhance aerobic fitness as well as bone density because of its weight-bearing characteristic. The best thing about walking is that it is an independent and inexpensive activity. You don't need a partner or a team, but you can just as easily work with a group, or even family members or friends.

Walking involves a rhythmic, forward action of the legs that targets the large lower muscles of the body including the hip flexors, gluteus maximus, quadriceps, and hamstrings. Assisting those muscles are the gastrocnemius and the anterior tibialis. The less obvious, but equally important, muscles are the hip abductors and hip adductors; these are responsible for stabilizing the hips and legs in general. The torso muscles are also actively engaged to keep your torso erect as you naturally swing your arms back and forth. Because walking is a major function of our lives, by engaging in this activity, we are training for real-life muscle function!

A well-fitted walking shoe is the most basic requirement for walking efficiently and safely. You will need to try on a variety of models to see which style provides the best overall fit. Because the greatest loads (sometimes your entire body weight) are at the heel and ball of the foot, choose a shoe that provides the most cushioning in both areas. The heel cup of the shoe should be stable and offer lateral (side-to-side) support as the heel contacts the ground. As you walk, your toes bend naturally and extend as you push off through your stride. Walking shoes need to be flexible enough in the forefoot to allow this to happen. A bevel (angle) in the heel of a walking shoe permits the smooth rolling motion of a walking gait. A nonbeveled heel will cause the toes to "slap" down rapidly, possibly causing shin soreness. Finally, the walking motion causes the foot and toes to spread, so allow for ample room in the toe box.

The mechanics of walking, especially when exercising, are quite distinct from the mechanics of other activities. Although any recreational shoe is appropriate for casual walking, choosing a performance walking shoe is a good idea if you will be walking for fitness because it is designed specifically for fitness walking, in the same way a running shoe is designed for running.

Typically there are three categories of walking: leisure or health walking, fitness walking, and speed or power walking. Although the movement processes in each category are similar, the execution techniques differ. Choose the technique that will work best for your goal of maintaining, enhancing, or increasing your cardiorespiratory system.

Leisure or Health Walking

As its name implies, leisure or health walking takes place at a normal, leisurely pace. At this pace a person would complete 1 mile (1.6 kilometers) in 16 to 30 minutes. This walking category, which is designed for the maintenance of cardiovascular endurance, is appropriate for anyone, especially those who are just starting a regular exercise walking program. Regular participation in leisure or health walking will reduce the risk of heart disease, lower the risk of osteoporosis, reduce body fat, and enhance feelings of well-being.

The most important component of leisure or health walking (and exercise in general) is good posture. Proper body alignment forms the mechanical foundation for safe and effective walking and allows you to function and perform efficiently. Focus your awareness on maintaining a tall, vertical, and erect posture with secondary emphasis on a natural and comfortable arm and leg action. Your chest should be lifted or expanded. Imagine being pulled up by a string attached to your sternum. Your abdominal muscles should be gently contracted throughout the walk. Imagine your navel being pulled gently toward your spine as your spine moves gently toward your navel. This will allow for a simultaneous contraction between the abdominal and back muscles to keep your torso erect and enhance your core strength through stabilization. Your arm swing should be natural and comfortable, and your elbows should be relaxed as your arms swing in opposition to your legs (see figure 4.1). The forward swing of your arms should never cross the center of your body. Allow your arms to swing close to the sides of your body. The length of each stride should be comfortable.

Most people adapt quickly to the demands of leisure or health walking. Once you have achieved a desired level of endurance with a leisure or health walking technique, you are ready to move up to the next level, fitness walking, if your goal is to increase fitness levels further. Fitness walking and speed walking (discussed next) have been specifically designed for improving cardiovascular endurance.

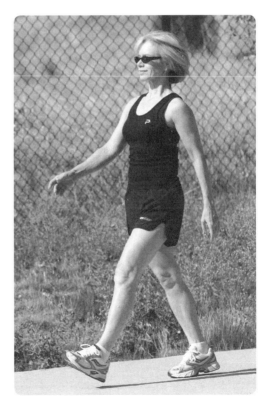

FIGURE 4.1   Correct form for leisure or health walking.

Fitness Walking

Like leisure or health walking, fitness walking is easily accessible. However, the objective of this walking style is to increase your aerobic fitness level, improve the condition of your heart and lungs, and expend more energy by burning more calories. To accomplish this, you will need to walk at pace of 13 to 15 minutes a mile (1.6 kilometers), which is a bit faster than in leisure or health walking. You need to be completely comfortable and successful with the intensity and techniques of leisure or health walking before moving to this intensity level.

A leisure or health walk becomes a fitness walk when you increase your speed by increasing the number of steps you take per minute. By increasing your speed rather than your stride, you will be able to maintain good form and alignment. The goal is to increase your cardiovascular endurance and remain aerobic; your intensity level should increase to the point at which you become more aware of your breathing, but are not breathless. The faster you bring your rear leg forward, the faster your rate of walking will be.

To increase the intensity of your walk, you may still wish to increase your stride. If you do increase your stride, be aware that an increase in stride tends to produce a forward lean. Take note of this on your walk and allow the lean to occur from your ankles and not your waist. Too much forward flexion or bending from the hips can lead to pain and discomfort in the lumbar area of your spine.

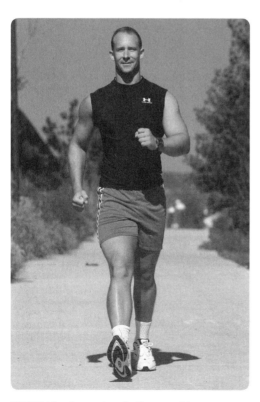

At this intensity level, your arm action will increase and your elbows will automatically begin to flex. The flexed elbow is a result of a faster stride so that the arms can maintain a faster swing. A faster arm swing will, in turn, cause an increase in your stride frequency. Be sure to allow the movement of your arms to come from your shoulders, not your elbows. Avoid swinging your arms from side to side like windshield wipers (with your elbows close to your body and your forearms hanging and swinging low across the center of your body). Your arms should move in opposition to your legs. The goal is to produce a smooth and fluid gait as a result of a natural rotation of the hips. The heel plant should allow for your forefoot and toes to be raised toward your shins. Your forefoot is then lowered to the ground with control to avoid slapping or pounding. Your foot should roll from heel to toe. See figure 4.2 for correct fitness walking form.

FIGURE 4.2　Correct form for fitness walking.

Speed or Race Walking

Speed or race walking is a form of walking for people looking for a greater physical challenge and a way to increase their caloric expenditure. This highly stylized technique is characterized by an obvious hip rotation that takes place as a result of the increased stride rate. It requires a high level of conditioning because the goal is to work at a pace of 12 minutes per mile (1.6 kilometers), which is 4 minutes faster than the fastest pace in leisure or health walking. Extremely skilled competitive walkers are known to walk at speeds between 9 and 10 miles per hour (between 14 and 16 kilometers per hour), which is a pace of 6 or 7 minutes per mile (1.6 kilometers). This is an impressive pace even for a runner.

At this quicker pace, a strong mastery of speed or race walking technique is needed to increase the stride frequency. To gain a clearer understanding, consider that in running, stride length plays a significant role when attempting to increase speed. However, in walking, stride length is limited because one foot is always in contact with the ground. To compensate for the faster action, the hip has to increase its rotation to increase stride frequency. To walk at this pace requires significant skill and technique development.

In speed or race walking, the arm position is the same as that of fitness walking. The elbows are flexed at about 90 degrees. As your arm swings forward, it should cross closer to the center of your body and swing no higher than your sternum. During the backswing, your hand should not reach farther than the back of your buttocks. Consciously drive your elbows back and keep them close to the sides of your body. Increasing the speed of your arm swing will increase your stride frequency. To increase your stride length, think of pulling your legs forward more quickly from your hips. Concentrate on increasing stride frequency rather than stride length. Feel your abdominal muscles and hip flexors initiate the quick forward pull of your leg as you roll off your toes. As your right leg swings forward, your supporting or left leg should remain straight. Be aware of the hip rotation that takes place as a result of this increased pace. Your hips should rotate forward and backward with a minimum of side-to-side motion. You will feel and notice the hip of your advancing leg tilt down as your leg reaches maximum forward rotation. This is where the "stylized action" comes from.

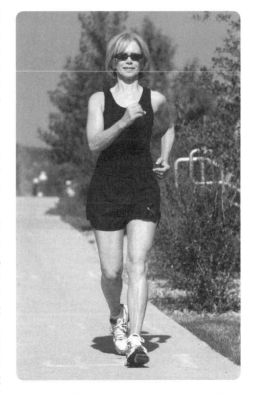

FIGURE 4.3 Correct form for speed or race walking. The placement of each foot should form a continuous straight line.

Because speed or race walking is a low-impact activity, concentrate on keeping the ball of your foot on the ground until the heel of your forward leg has contacted the ground. As in all forms of walking, you should roll smoothly from your heel to the ball of your foot with a strong push-off from the ball of your foot. However, at these higher walking speeds, the placement of the foot should form a continuous straight line, with the inner edge of one foot landing in front of the inner edge of the other foot (see figure 4.3). Imagine that you are walking on a tightrope with the inner edges of each foot landing on either side of the tightrope. As in fitness walking, lean slightly forward from your ankles. This slight forward lean will give you a feeling of being able to push against the ground harder, helping to maintain your correct stride length.

Jogging

Jogging is the next natural step from walking. Jogging is a form of trotting or running at a slow or leisurely pace with the main intention to increase fitness, endurance, and caloric expenditure. Jogging, like walking, can be done anytime, anywhere, and can be done alone or in a group. Jogging has all the health benefits of walking: It conditions the heart, improves muscle tone and strength, relieves stress, and can help with a variety of health problems including heart disease and arthritis. However, whereas walking is a low-impact activity because one foot is always in contact with the ground, in jogging and in running, impact is introduced. This is a high-impact exercise that places strain on the body, notably the joints of the knee. But impact can actually be a good thing. Because jogging is a weight-bearing activity, it will enhance bone density, which can reduce the risk of osteoporosis.

The big advantage of jogging over walking is that you can cover the same distance in a shorter period of time. The disadvantage is that it can result in more injuries than walking, because the strain placed on both muscles and joints is greater. But with proper shoes and preparation through stretching, you can greatly reduce your risk of injury.

Jogging and running, like walking, involve rhythmic, forward action of the legs that target the large lower muscles of the body including the hip flexors, gluteus maximus, quadriceps, and hamstrings. Assisting those muscles are the gastrocnemius and the anterior tibialis. The less obvious, yet equally important, muscles are your hip abductors and hip adductors, which are responsible for stabilizing the hips and legs in general. The torso muscles are also actively engaged to keep your torso erect as your arms swing naturally with your stride. Because of the level of impact associated with both jogging and running, proper alignment of the torso is paramount in limiting stress to the joints and low back. Visualize and create a tall vertical position of your torso, keeping your abdominal muscles engaged throughout your jog. Maintain a strong upper postural position by keeping your shoulders down, creating lots of distance between your shoulders and ears to avoid carrying your arms too high.

While jogging, you should leap, transferring your weight evenly and softly from one foot to the next (see figure 4.4). You should avoid leaping too high into the air, however, and landing heavily on your heel. Such form wastes energy and exacerbates the impact of the exercise. Create a normal foot strike that lands flat on the outer back portion of the heel, rolls onto the sole, and ends with the push-off from the ball of the foot. A heavy heel strike can lead to excessive traumatic forces and actually slow you down. Landing on the midfoot or ball of the foot places more stress on the Achilles tendon (which contracts to counterbalance the force of the strike).

A well-fitted running shoe is the most basic requirement for jogging. You will need to try on a variety of models to see which style provides the best overall fit. The amount of cushioning you require depends on how hard your foot strikes the ground

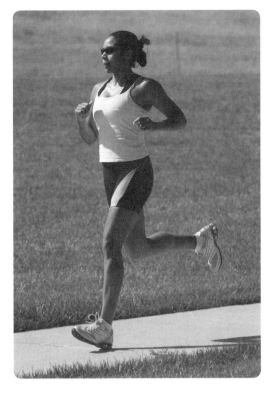

FIGURE 4.4 Correct jogging form. The foot strike should be soft.

during your stride. The frame and build of your body will help you determine how much cushioning you need. A small-framed person does not create a severe impact with the ground in comparison to a large-framed person, and so would require less overall cushioning. Because the greatest loads are at the heel and ball of the foot (as much as three times your body weight), choose a shoe that provides the most cushioning in both areas. The heel cup of the shoe should be stable and offer lateral (side-to-side) support as your heel contacts the ground. As you jog, your toes bend and extend as you push off through your stride. Running shoes need to be flexible enough in the forefoot to allow this to happen. The jogging motion also causes the foot and toes to spread, so allow for ample room in the toe box. Most experts agree that a good pair of comfortable sneakers will suffice; however, as we recommended in walking, choosing a well constructed performance running shoe is a good idea because it is designed specifically for running and will help you avoid injury. If you take the time to choose proper footwear, your feet will not only perform better, they'll feel better too!

All in all, jogging is an efficient and effective way to maintain or enhance your level of cardiovascular fitness. It is also the perfect preparation for running, the next intensity level of high-impact activity for your morning cardio workout.

Running

Running is one of the most popular forms of exercise in the world because virtually anyone can do it. It is my activity of choice! People begin running for a lot of reasons. Many want to lose weight, some do so to complement their athletic endeavors, and others begin as a recommendation from their physicians or specialists to strengthen the muscles in their feet and legs. And then there are those who do it for the sheer enjoyment of the activity, almost as a form of meditation, an opportunity to focus and get into themselves. Many runners derive benefits beyond the physical. Those runners and joggers who run longer distances (greater than 20 minutes) often experience a release of endorphins, more commonly referred to as a "runner's high." This feeling of euphoria acts as a stress release to some and a form of meditation to others. The benefits of running can be mental as well as physical. This holds true for walkers as well.

The physical movements of running are identical to those of jogging, only they are done faster. Running is the next logical progression from jogging if you are looking to enhance caloric expenditure and cardiorespiratory fitness. Running burns more calories than jogging because of its higher intensity, so you will consume more oxygen in the long run. More oxygen consumed translates to more calories burned. According to the American Council on Exercise (2003), a 160-pound (73-kilogram) person running at 6 miles (9.6 kilometers) per hour can burn about 125 calories each minute. Carrying more body weight or increasing your speed will burn more calories for the same amount of exercise time, whereas carrying less body weight or decreasing your speed will burn less.

Like jogging, running is associated with a number of health benefits, the most important of which is strengthening the heart and lungs. The advantage of running over jogging is that it takes less time. The fact that running burns more calories also makes this an activity ideal for weight management, if that is among your goals. Running shares the same disadvantages of jogging because of the high impact level, which can lead to more joint injuries. But with proper shoes and preparation through training and stretching, you can greatly reduce this risk. See the jogging section for how to select proper running footwear.

The physical movements of running are virtually identical to those of jogging. It involves a rhythmic, forward action of the legs that targets the large lower muscles of the body including the gluteus maximus, hip flexors, quadriceps, hamstrings, gastrocnemius, and anterior tibialis. In both running and jogging, the hamstrings and gastrocnemius tend to get the greatest use because of the impact that occurs as the heel strikes the ground. The heel strike allows for the calf to stretch, reducing the stress to that area as well as to the Achilles tendon and promotes better shock absorption. The hip adductors and abductors are involved the way they are in jogging, to stabilize the legs and allow for proper gait. When you maintain the correct posture and alignment, your entire core (abdominal, back, and upper postural muscles) benefit because they are required to stabilize your torso.

Upper postural stabilization is also important in running, as we discussed in jogging. Allowing your arms to swing back and forth naturally and avoiding holding them too high will allow for a more efficient workout. You should land on your heels, not on the balls of your feet. Your heel should hit the ground first, and then your arch should come down, followed by the ball of your foot and your toes. You take off from the ball of your foot—and then you are into your next step. Landing on the balls of your feet is not recommended because your calf muscles will not get a chance to stretch but will remain in a contracted state, contributing to tight calves. Although any form of running will make your calf muscle shorter, running on the balls of your feet will actually make this condition worse (although it may help you run faster).

When encountering a hill or incline, allow the forward lean of your body to come from your ankle joints rather than your hips or waist (see figure 4.5). This technique will allow you to maintain your stride and keep your torso erect. When approaching a decline, lean back slightly (see figure 4.6). The degree of your lean should be based on the degree of the decline. Stay focused and centered to maintain your vertical position when running downhill. With a faster pace comes an increase in the frequency of the swinging action of your arms. Your arms should not cross your midline or move to the front of your body as though you were rocking a baby. Keep them by your sides and allow them to swing naturally in opposition to your legs.

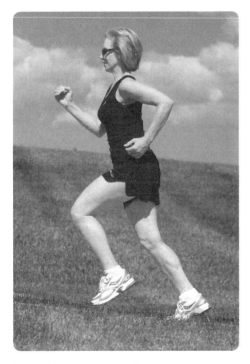

FIGURE 4.5   Running on an incline.

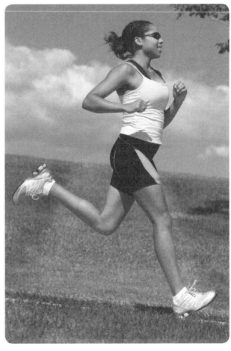

FIGURE 4.6   Running on a decline.

A major consideration should be where to run safely. Having a running partner is best to remain safe. Many areas have running clubs that offer regular group runs, which is a great way to network and find running partners. Surfaces should be taken into consideration as well, for the safety of your joints and muscles. Blacktop is more forgiving than concrete. Dirt and wood chip pathways tend to be more scenic and allow for more cushioning on the joints. A typical runner takes 1,500 steps per mile, or 900 steps per kilometer! This can be very stressful on the joints of the body, considering that each time you land, almost three times the amount of your body weight is placed on your joints. Running on softer surfaces and stretching after your run can be helpful in reducing the risk of injuries to your knees, shins, ankles, and low back.

Cycling

Did you know that there are over 33 million adult cyclists in the United States? And that number continues to grow at the recreational level. Interest in cycling has grown as a result of an increased interest in cardiovascular exercise. Many people are looking for an aerobic activity that is nonimpact and familiar; cycling meets these criteria because it is an activity that many people learn in their youth. In addition, with fluctuating fuel prices and growing environmental conscious- ness, cycling has become an alternative to motor transportation. The bicycle is a tremendously efficient means of transportation. In fact, cycling is more efficient than any other method of travel—including walking! The human body is the efficient fuel.

Everyday cycling that leaves you breathing heavily but not out of breath is an effective and enjoyable form of aerobic exercise. Cycling reduces the risk of serious conditions such as heart disease, high blood pressure, obesity, and the most common form of diabetes. Like most aerobic activities, cycling will also help with weight management through caloric expenditure. It is a muscle-specific activity, primarily focusing on the quadriceps and hamstrings and allowing for increases in leg strength while improving cardiovascular fit- ness. Working the legs also enhances hip mobility, which can help improve your performance of everyday activities. In general, cycling is a great way to strengthen the muscles of the lower body that we use to get through the daily physical stresses of life.

Most cyclists also assert that cycling not only improves their physical health but also has a positive effect on how they feel. A sense of accomplishment and a feeling of independence and freedom are feelings most cyclists share. Perhaps that's why cycling for many is more than a sport or even a mode of transporta- tion—it's a passion. Finally, outdoor cycling can allow you to meditate and get in touch with nature. Cycling outdoors is a great way to observe the scenery of the land around you, allowing you to take in the beauty of nature while you improve your fitness levels.

Cycling is a nonimpact activity and so is a great alternative to walking or running. The pedaling action of the lower body creates a push and pull action of the quadriceps, hamstrings, and ankle joints. The goal is to create smooth, synchronized movements of the feet and the legs so that the feet "spin" in an efficient circular motion that follows the pedal rotation. The foot, lower leg, thigh, and pelvis act as a set of jointed levers, and the muscles provide the forces that cause the ankle, knee, and hip joints to flex and extend. The force the muscle can exert varies with its length; the stronger the riders are, the more force they can apply.

When cycling, keep your abdominal and back extensor muscles engaged and maintain a strong and stable base in the shoulder area, keeping your shoulders pressed down away from your ears. Imagining that you are sliding your shoulders down toward your back pockets is a helpful visualization. Your hands and wrists should remain in a neutral position; avoid gripping the handlebars too tightly. Keep your knees tracking forward over your feet, being careful not to allow your knees to waver from side to side. Your toes should disappear from sight at the bottom of the stroke.

Cycling equipment today varies greatly. With many styles and so many prices, how do you know which is best for you? The choices can be overwhelming. A good, professional bike shop is usually the best source of information. Before going bike shopping, you need to define yourself a bit and consider where and how you will pedal. Will you be primarily riding on the road, or will you primarily work in parks and on trails? Are you looking for a bike that will support your back? Will you look to challenge yourself by racing? Later in this section, we describe three common types of biking. The activity you choose will determine the bike you need. Once you choose your activity, a professional bike shop will help you choose the appropriate bike.

In cycling, safety and prevention are key, and certain equipment is necessary. It is important to take the necessary precautions to prevent injury and make this exhilarating mode of exercise safe. Head injuries and other injuries related to accidents are the most common that occur in cycling. A helmet designed to absorb the force of impact is recommended to avoid head injuries during a fall. It should be close fitting and not pushed too far back on the head. Bicycles should be equipped with front, side, and rear reflectors. Cyclists who ride at dusk or night should also wear reflective clothing.

Footwear is another important piece of cycling equipment. Although cycling can be done in a casual recreational shoe, taking the time to obtain proper cycling shoes can make a huge difference in your riding. Cycling shoes have stiff soles to help transfer power from your feet to the pedals as well as to protect your feet. Sneakers with soft soles can allow your arches to collapse while pedaling which can cause pain and tendon problems as well as a burning sensation on the bottom of your feet. Cycling shoes should have a snug fit so your feet don't move around. They have special fixing points for cleats that attach the shoe to the pedals. If you are using a recreational shoe, be sure that it is flexible in the ball of the foot rather than bending at the center so the power is generated to the front part of the foot while pedaling.

There are three main types of cycling: road cycling, recumbent cycling, and race cycling. Each requires a specific type of bike and has unique components and considerations.

Road Cycling

A road bike is built for use on pavement and is perfect for commutes, fitness, or leisure riding and touring. Many people choose road cycling for the pure enjoyment of exploring new trails, being outside with nature, and enjoying the cardiovascular benefits of endurance riding. For the most part, the amount of conditioning this activity yields depends on the length and intensity of the ride. You could take a leisurely ride and work at a comfortable level, or you could ride along a long and winding road to enhance cardiovascular endurance as you take in the beauty of the scenery. Those bitten by the cycling bug may choose to take long rides, covering 30 to 50 miles (48 to 80 kilometers) a day, further enhancing their fitness levels. Road cycling is an excellent way to enhance cardiovascular endurance, leg strength, and overall physical conditioning.

Road cycling involves an upright posture while your lower body performs the pedaling action to move the bike (see figure 4.7). This forces your abdominal

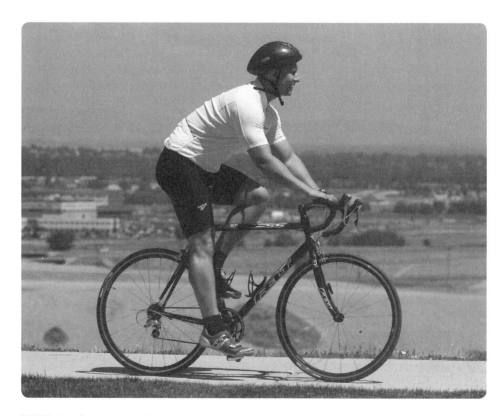

FIGURE 4.7   Correct road cycling posture.

muscles and back extensors (the stabilizing muscles of the torso) to contract to keep your body upright. Your arms should be fully extended, and you should have a light grip on the handlebars.

For a challenging workout, choose a route that involves inclines and rolling hills. This will increase the intensity of the ride allowing for more caloric expenditure and create more of an interval effect to the ride. The bursts of energy required to cycle uphill will help you gain leg strength as well as the ability to cycle at higher intensities for longer periods of time, thereby enhancing your stamina and overall fitness level. For best performance, your posture should adjust to whether you are riding uphill or downhill. Riding uphill will require a change in position to access more of the hamstrings to help power you through the climb. Your torso will flex forward more; you should hinge from the hips and not be rounded at the shoulders. This position will force your torso stabilizers to work to maintain this strong, stable posture as you pedal harder. You may want to shift your weight back on the seat a bit as you climb or ride against strong wind to access more of the hamstrings and gluteals. Your hands should be in the extended position on the handlebars, fingers relaxed, not gripping.

Check your community paper or search online to find scenic trails and routes in your area. This is the safest way to ride rather than daring the busy streets where numerous stop signs interrupt your ride. You might also find charity rides that are both noncompetitive and fun.

Recumbent Cycling

Comfort is key to this type of cycling. With a recumbent bike, which resembles a lawn chair on wheels, you are in a reclined position with a backrest to support your low back so your whole upper body is relaxed above your hips. The seat is usually a little larger, which allows for more comfort in riding. The lower center of gravity makes for better balance as well. Recumbent cycling is recommended for those with back problems because of the back support offered by the seat. It is ideal for those with conditions such as arthritis, or for those who need comfort in aerobic exercise. But don't let the position fool you; like upright cycling, it offers a sufficient cardiovascular workout. Recumbent cycling qualifies as an excellent cross-training activity to add to your morning workout regimen. Because it recruits different actions of the hamstrings and quadriceps and challenges your balance capabilities, it adds variety to your training regimen.

The structure of a recumbent bike is different from that of a road bike, and so it requires a modified posture. Your legs will perform the same pedaling action as with road biking, but the action will come more from the hamstrings than from the quadriceps because of the reclining position. Your arms extend out in front of your body and are held a little higher than they are in road biking. Upper-body stabilization is important here, so keep your shoulders down and away from your ears while maintaining an upright and erect posture. It is easy to get lazy and lean against the backrest, letting your torso just "hang out." Instead of doing that, stay focused on keeping your abdominal and back extensor muscles engaged to force the stabilizing muscles to work to maintain your torso in an erect position. (See figure 4.8.) Because the position is a bit different from that in road biking, it would be best to practice in an area free of traffic, such as a large open parking lot, to perfect your technique and balance. Once confident, you can head for the road and trails where you can experience a variety of terrain and get to your destination in comfort while enjoying the moment.

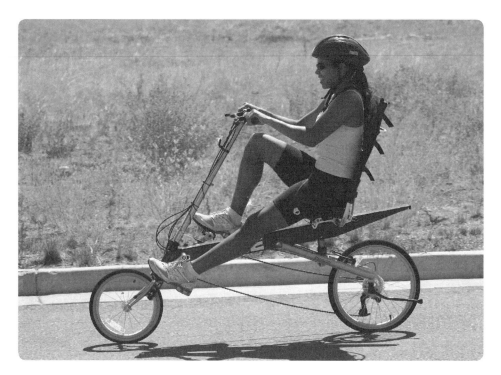

FIGURE 4.8   Correct recumbent biking posture.

Race Cycling

A racing bike is the ultimate in efficiency; it is lightweight and designed for those who ride fast and hard on the pavement. If you are competitive in nature, then race cycling may be a good choice for adding variety to your cycling or morning workouts. Whether your preference is to race against other cyclists or against the clock, race cycling is a technique that requires a strong foundation of cycling before beginning. It is performed at an intensity level that will elicit a higher cardiorespiratory response than road or recumbent cycling, because increased speed and power is the goal.

Because the rate of pedaling is a learned response, drills that encourage increased pedal speed should be introduced into your normal workouts before beginning race cycling. Drills such as "spin-ups," in which cadence is progressively increased at regular intervals at a moderate resistance, as well as "surges," in which gradual, controlled increases in cadence are performed while riding at a moderately high to high resistance, usually in a climb, will prepare you for the increased demands of racing.

Muscles involved in race cycling are the same as described in the main cycling section, with the quadriceps, hamstrings, and gluteals being the main source of power. The pumping, pedaling action of the legs is consistent with that of road biking; however, it is the fast rate of pedaling that is characteristic here. The faster you can turn the pedals, the more ground you will cover in the shortest amount of time. You will need to adapt technique and form for the most efficient pedal stroke when racing. Typically, racing is performed with a fast cadence (or high pedaling rate) on a surface with little resistance, such as flat terrain, as speed is the emphasis. This can be done seated or standing, the latter usually used to sprint to the finish line. The sitting position is more upright with the "sitz bones" pressing into the saddle when seated. Hips are hinged, yet the torso remains lifted. Abdominal muscles and back extensors are engaged. The knees are slightly bent when the pedal is bottom center. Pedals are typically parallel to the ground (see figure 4.9*a*). When lifting off the saddle, position your hips over the saddle while maintaining a strong neutral alignment of your pelvis and torso (see figure 4.9*b*).

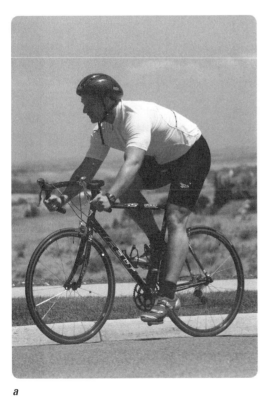 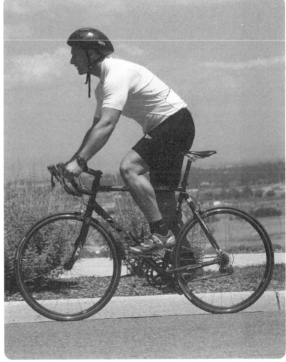

a *b*

FIGURE 4.9   Correct racing cycle form: *(a)* seated, *(b)* standing.

Bicycle racing can be an individual or team effort. You don't have to be an elite cyclist to race, either. A lot of communities and organizations have beginner clinics to help get you started in this fast-paced, exhilarating sport. In these clinics you will learn strategies to be more competitive, rules, scoring, etiquette, nutrition, hydration, sprint workouts, riding in a group, bike maintenance, and what to expect on race day. There are also numerous race cycling clubs throughout the United States and internationally. Joining a club in your area is a great way to meet people with the same interests, learn more about cycling, join a team and race with others, and keep up the internal motivation to succeed and win.

5

Indoor Activities

Does this sound like your day? Up at 6 a.m., make coffee, jump into the shower, get dressed and ready for work, get the kids up, make breakfast. Then, organize lunches or daily errands, get the kids dressed, walk the dog, shuffle the kids to the babysitter or bus, run out the door to work—you barely have enough time to eat yourself, let alone exercise! Considering the fast-paced society we now live in and how much we have to pack into one day, the need for time-efficient, convenient ways to exercise is paramount. Although exercising outdoors allows you to get outside, sometimes inclement weather combined with the craziness of your day doesn't leave enough time to prepare for an outdoor activity. Exercising indoors at home or at a fitness facility gives you a plethora of options to get your workout done without dealing with the weather and gives the wonderful opportunity to cross-train and actually perform two or more modes of exercise in one session if you choose.

This chapter discusses a variety of indoor workout options. Although indoor workouts can be performed without any machines, today there are numerous types of machines designed to replicate cardiovascular activities from walking to skating, with intensity options that can match most of the intensity variables you face outside. You can achieve the same health and cardiovascular benefits indoors as you can outdoors.

All of the options we describe in this chapter are readily available at your local health or fitness facility. A representative at your club can guide you through the operation of each piece of equipment you are unfamiliar with. A health club membership, proper footwear, your MP3 player, a towel if the club does not provide them, and water are all you need to get you through your workout.

If working at home is more convenient for you, you have many options as well. Most commercial-grade machine manufacturers offer residential models of the equipment you find in health clubs. These models are less expensive than commercial models and can still be of high quality. If many people in the family will be using a machine in your home gym, however, you may want to consider a commercial-grade model, which is built to withstand multiple users every day. Having exercise equipment in your home offers the convenience of keeping your workout on track on the days you can't get outside or to the gym.

Also addressed in this chapter are indoor water workouts. Water exercise is a great way to work your heart and increase your muscular strength. Moving your body through the water increases the intensity of your workout by using the resistance of the water. The water activities explored here can actually be done either inside *or* outside. However, because many health clubs and recreational facilities offer indoor pools, we have included them in this indoor section to make water exercise a year-round activity.

Treadmills

The treadmill is probably the most popular piece of exercise equipment in the gym today. During the morning hours it is not unusual to see every treadmill in a gym or fitness facility in use. This is a great way to increase cardiovascular endurance, increase speed, and improve balance. Treadmill exercise is essentially walking, jogging, or running in place. It allows you to take your walking or running program inside where you can maintain the pace of your stride. The mechanics used in walking, jogging, and running can all be applied here. The difference is that you are not going anywhere.

When you are walking or running on a treadmill, the major muscles in motion are the quadriceps, hamstrings, and gluteals, as well as the gastrocnemius (large calf muscle), anterior tibialis (shin muscle), and ankle joint. As in all upright activities, the abdominal muscles and back extensors are involved to keep your torso erect, and the hip abductors and adductors are involved to keep your gait solid. The advantage of walking or running on a treadmill is that you are typically on a cushioned surface. This lessens the impact on the joints in comparison to walking or running on concrete or black asphalt. A treadmill platform is more flexible and has higher shock absorption than outdoor running surfaces, so if you have trouble with your knees or hips, running on a treadmill can be the best option for you.

A lot of workout options are available when working out on a treadmill. Most treadmills have speed and incline variables offering you the opportunity to vary your intensity throughout your routine. You can simulate outdoor workouts and add challenge or modification to your workout by using these variables. These options allow you to work toward your conditioning goals while enhancing your cardiovascular response and burning calories. You can also do interval conditioning on a treadmill, setting up rest periods at lower intensities between high-intensity bouts of exercise. Interval conditioning is a great way to train your body to work at higher intensities for longer periods of time to increase your cardiovascular performance and burn more calories in the long run. See chapter 6 for a more complete discussion of interval conditioning.

The following guidelines will you help keep proper form during your treadmill workout and get the most out of your routine. See figure 5.1 for a photo of the correct full-body technique.

- **Footwork.** As your foot comes forward and your heel strikes the platform, raise your toes and roll forward onto the outside of your foot (but keep the entire shoe sole on the platform). As your foot passes under your body, straighten your knee and press down on the platform with the ball of your foot, maintaining pressure until your toes leave the platform.

- **Hip movement.** Allow your hips to rotate naturally with the forward and backward movement of your legs. Concentrate on keeping your shoulders relaxed and facing forward.

- **Arm swing.** Let your arms swing naturally by your sides in opposition to your legs in the same forward and backward direction as your hips and legs. When increasing speed, bend your arms at a slight right angle and swing them faster in rhythm with your legs.

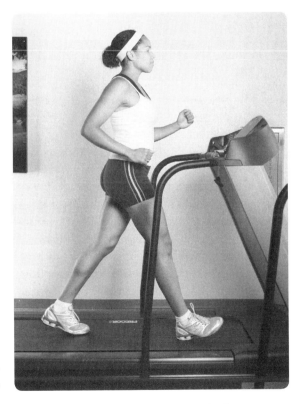

When you first try a treadmill, you may find your balance challenged as a result of the movement of the belt. It is important to start by holding onto the treadmill handles. As you gain confidence and your balance improves, you can let go and move your arms as though you were walking down the street. Start with walking and work on increasing speed on a flat surface until you feel comfortable with the speed and balance. This will allow your muscles' proprioceptors (sensors that detect the various forces placed on the body) to prepare for the increases in speed and incline that you choose to implement.

FIGURE 5.1   Proper treadmill walking or running form.

Walking on a treadmill feels a little awkward at first, but keep your stride length and heel strike the same as you would if you were walking on the ground. Be careful that you don't set the speed too fast at first or you could fall off of the back of the treadmill. All treadmills come with a safety strap that you can clip to your shirt. This will automatically stop the treadmill if you should ever fall. After you are finished with your first workout on a treadmill, stop the treadmill, hold onto the rails, and stand still for a couple of minutes until you feel your equilibrium return. Some people feel a little light-headed until they get used to the motion of walking in one place.

Treadmill exercise is convenient, effective, and efficient. You can work out at your own pace, weather isn't a problem, and, with a variety training options available (as we will share with you in later chapters), neither is boredom. Put on your walking or running shoes and get moving!

Elliptical Trainers

Tired of the treadmill? Looking for an alternative to cycling? Are you in the market for a cardiovascular workout that gets you in shape without being hard on your knees? Then elliptical machines may be ideal for you. Elliptical trainers offer a low-impact workout that is easy on the joints and still gives you the feeling of working your entire body. Ellipticals are appropriate for all fitness levels and are a great way to improve your cross-training workout while burning as many calories as you would burn using a treadmill or cross-country ski machine. They add variety and keep you motivated if you get bored with your current fitness routine.

The best advantage of an elliptical trainer is the motion it creates. The elliptical motion simulates walking, stepping, cycling, and skiing using an elliptical motion to deliver various combinations of workouts. In most cases, because both feet are primarily in contact with the pedals at all times, the workout can be classified as nonimpact, making this a workout with minimal impact on the joints of the body. Combine that with the ability to offer a reverse action of the foot pedals, and the elliptical is in a class by itself. Some models offer dual-action handlebars, allowing you to incorporate your upper body. If your machine has arm handles and you've achieved proper balance, you can pump the arms in the same way you would when you walk to burn extra calories. Models with or without arm handles allow you to adjust the incline to increase your caloric expenditure. With elliptical trainers you can work on cardiovascular endurance or intervals just as you can on a treadmill.

Elliptical machines, like treadmills, are very popular at the club level. However, commercial manufacturers offer home versions at affordable prices that allow you to work out in the convenience of your home. Like the commercial models, the home models come in versions that include motions solely for the lower body or that offer arm handles to incorporate your upper body into the workout. The variety of options allows you to choose the machine that will work best for you in helping you achieve your goals.

With the elliptical trainer simulating a variety of motions, the quadriceps, hamstrings, gastrocnemius, anterior tibialis, and the ankle joint are all involved in this process. When the handlebars are used, the deltoids (shoulder muscles), latissimus dorsi (back muscles), biceps, and triceps become involved as well. Torso muscles are activated as the abdominal muscles and back extensors simultaneously contract to keep you in the upright position, and the upper postural muscles are engaged to support the action of the arms. This provides the perfect environment to enhance torso stabilization while maintaining proper form and alignment.

Used correctly, elliptical trainers offer a challenging and effective low-impact workout and are a great alternative to running, especially because they put less pressure on the knees and hips. See figure 5.2 for proper form while using an elliptical trainer. To ensure proper form, follow guidelines from the manufacturer or your health club before using the machine

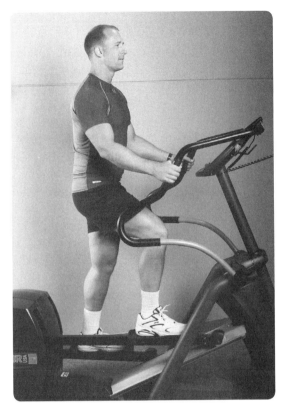

FIGURE 5.2   Proper form while using an elliptical trainer.

for the first time. Make sure your entire foot remains on the pedal and that you perform smooth pedal strokes with even strides and avoid bouncing through the pedal strokes. Shift your weight a bit back when in the reverse mode. Avoid leaning on or into the handlebars; instead, try to pedal as though you were not relying on them. Do not add weights because they may damage or interfere with your stride. Also make sure not to put too much resistance on the machine because it can cause strain to the knees. Wear a comfortable cross-training shoe that has good lateral support and room in the toe box. Extra cushioning is not necessary because this is primarily a low- or nonimpact activity.

Stair Steppers

If climbing is more your speed, then stair-stepping machines would be a good option for your morning cardio workout. Stair-stepping machines are one of the most popular pieces of fitness equipment in use for aerobic workouts today. The act of climbing for fitness is not new. For many years, athletic coaches and trainers have used the bleacher stands in stadiums as well as flights of stairs to condition their athletes. Some reviews indicate that elliptical trainers have taken over the stair-stepping market because the ski-type motion and incline of elliptical machines provide a greater variety of aerobic workout while limiting the impact on joints. However, stair steppers have proven to be effective because they provide a lower-impact aerobic workout than running, and stepping helps tone the lower-body muscle because you are lifting your body weight with each step that you take.

Stair steppers provide an aerobic workout by allowing you to create a climbing action by pushing independent foot pedals up and down, or in some models, by climbing a rotating staircase. Most models offer adjustable resistance and speed variables to vary intensity. The primary muscles used in stair climbing are the quadriceps, hip flexors, and hamstrings, assisted by the gastrocnemius, soleus (lower calf muscle), anterior tibialis, and ankle joint. The hip flexors have to flex and extend as you push the pedals down to create the climbing action. This climbing action is what promotes the increased cardiorespiratory response, while also increasing muscular strength.

Correct posture is paramount in stair stepping (see figure 5.3). Maintain an upright and stable position with your abdominal muscles and back extensors engaged. Keep your chest lifted and avoid leaning forward and putting all your weight onto your arms, because doing so will defeat the purpose of a great lower-body workout and can strain your back and neck. Some models offer upright handles located above the display to help you stay upright. Make use of these when you feel fatigued, but again, avoid leaning onto them. Reduce your intensity so that you can maintain the upright posture on your own with minimal assistance. Keep enough resistance on the stair stepper so that you can control your stepping motion and not rock your pelvis from side to side. Keep your feet flat on the pedals and work within a range that is comfortable without compromising your alignment. Be careful not to bottom out on the pedals. The higher the levels, the faster the pedals move, so the faster you have to move your body to keep up with the machine. Maintaining your correct posture throughout this intensity change is important to gain the most positive benefits. You should wear a pair of comfortable cross-training shoes that offer stable lateral support. Cushioning will help, but because this is a nonimpact activity, it is not the main focus.

Stair stepping is a great way to prepare your body for other activities as well. If you enjoy hiking and rock climbing, the action of stair stepping can help you prepare for the demands of those activities while also increasing and challenging your fitness level. It is truly a cardiovascular activity that can take you to new heights!

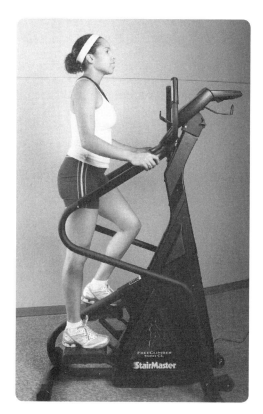

FIGURE 5.3   Correct stair-stepper posture.

Stationary Bikes

Is inclement weather getting in the way of your morning workout? Are you looking for a way to cross-train in a nonimpact activity? Are you in need of strengthening the muscles in your legs to enhance the integrity of your knees in addition to gaining cardiovascular endurance? Then the stationary bike may be the answer for you. Stationary bikes have been a staple in health clubs and facilities for years. In addition, they are a popular piece of equipment many have incorporated into their homes as well. Using the stationary bike is simple and nonintimidating because most people have cycled in their youth. Exercising on a stationary bike provides a gentle, yet effective low- or nonimpact workout without putting too much stress on the spine. This is a wonderful advantage to those who experience low back discomfort from time to time. In fact, physical therapists have incorporated stationary bikes into their practices for years in rehabbing knee injuries in athletes so that they can maintain their cardiovascular endurance. With most stationary bikes offering resistance variables, you have the ability to increase your aerobic fitness.

Riding a stationary bike strengthens the quadriceps and hamstrings and involves the use of the gastrocnemius, anterior tibialis, and ankle joint. Although stationary bikes do not specifically target the abs and back muscles, when cycling, you do have to keep your body in the upright, vertical position to maintain alignment of the pelvis and prevent hyperextension of the back. Riding a bike, whether stationary or a road cycle, improves the flexibility of the leg muscles (especially the hamstrings), which further helps to reduce low back pain from muscle strain. The cycling action also helps maintain the range of motion and flexibility of the many joints in the spine and legs, which in turn aids in maintaining flexibility levels throughout the lower body.

As described in our cycling section in chapter 4, there are two components to the cycling stroke: pushing down on the pedal and pulling up on the pedal. Both strokes are equally important; pushing down on the pedal requires the use of the quadriceps, and as you continue through the pedal stroke, the hamstrings are engaged as the knee flexes to assist the upward action of the stroke. Visualize the foot going in a circular pattern, pushing on the downstroke and pulling up on the upstroke. Also, although a stationary bike may be more comfortable than an outdoor cycle or a stair stepper, it is important to concentrate on contracting your abdominal muscles as you ride. See figure 5.4 for proper stationary biking posture.

Stationary bikes usually have adjustable seats. Prior to your ride, adjust the height of your seat so that your extended leg has a slight bend when the pedals are flat. A seat that is too high will pull your pelvis out of alignment; a seat that is too low can put your knee in a compromising position as well as affect your pelvic and hip position. Aim for a smooth pedal stroke so that you can maintain an upright posture without bouncing uncontrollably in the saddle. A comfortable, recreational shoe that is flexible in the ball of the foot is all that is required for this activity. Some bikes have straps or toe cages to help keep your foot in place on the pedal. Cushioning is not an issue because impact is not an issue.

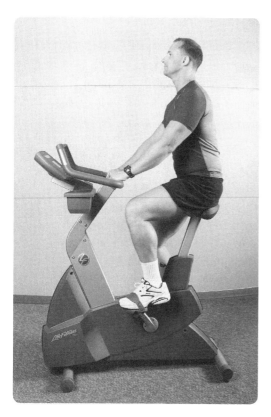

FIGURE 5.4   Proper stationary bike posture.

The key to effective and efficient cycling is to make sure that you maintain a good balance between resistance and the spinning of your legs. Because you are seated for the workout, you have to work harder to increase your heart rate and burn calories. You can increase your RPM (revolutions per minute), increase the resistance, or do both to maximize your workout. If you find yourself bouncing in the saddle, that is usually an indication that you do not have sufficient resistance on the bike. If this happens, increase your resistance a bit and slow your pedal stroke down to get the most out of your workout.

Spinning-type bikes, originally used for indoor group cycling classes, have become increasingly popular on the health club floor and in the home. These bikes are smaller and sleeker than traditional stationary bikes and look more like outdoor bikes. They have a fixed gear, racing handlebars, pedals equipped with clips or cages to accommodate cycling shoes, and adjustable seats. A spinning-type bike gives you the feeling of cycling outside and offer resistance options as well. You can stand as well as sit on the cycle, giving you a workout that can simulate an outdoor ride without the wind and other weather elements. These workouts give you the opportunity to take your cycling indoors and can provide an effective off-road training experience because you can perform most any technique that you would on an outdoor ride. A typical program led by a certified instructor lasts about 40 minutes.

You'll want to be sure to fit this type of bike to your height. Start by adjusting the height of the seat to the level of your hip bones. The seat can be adjusted fore and aft as well. Typically, the shorter your torso is, the more forward you should adjust your seat; the longer your torso is, the farther back you should position the seat.

Be sure to vary your resistance and use both sitting and standing positions to give yourself a well-rounded workout. (See figure 5.5 for proper sitting and standing positions.) When incorporating position changes, be sure to have enough resistance on the flywheel to support your standing position. As you increase your resistance levels, try moving your weight a bit farther back in the saddle to engage the hamstrings. This will help you vary the muscles you are using. Whether you ride a stationary bike or a spinning-type bike during your morning workout, a well-designed ride can give you an efficient workout in a short amount of time.

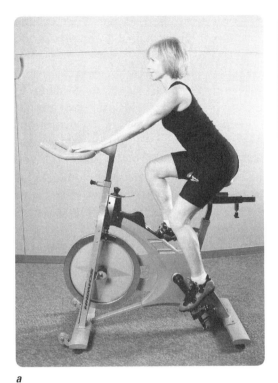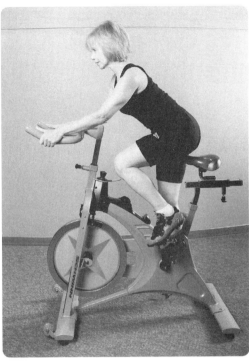

a

b

FIGURE 5.5   Correct posture on a spinning-type bike: *(a)* seated; *(b)* standing.

Rowing Machines

Picture this: gliding smoothly over glassy water, feeling the wind in your face as your heart pumps and your muscles contract rhythmically. Sound peaceful and appealing to you? Then rowing may be just the activity to give your morning cardio workout a boost. Whether you are actually on a lake or on a machine, rowing is a great exercise that benefits both the upper and lower body. It is invigorating and challenging at the same time. A rowing machine simulates rowing a boat with oars. This is great for toning your muscles while at the same time achieving your cardiovascular goals. It is a low-impact activity that consists of a smooth, rhythmic motion that prevents impact on your knees; as a result, it causes less joint problems in the long run. The rowing machine can dramatically increase your fitness levels because it engages many muscles and thus burns a substantial amount of calories. Some of the models even have water in the wheels to help increase the resistance and give you the sound of the waves so you can feel as though you are rowing down the river.

Rowing involves the gluteus maximus, quadriceps, hamstrings, and the muscles of the lower legs. The upper-body muscles involved include the upper back muscles, the trapezius and rhomboids as well as the biceps and triceps. It is a wonderful way to improve and condition your entire body in one workout. The technique of rowing, which mimics the action of driving a scull through water, is a multijoint activity that challenges the entire body.

You begin in the rest position, sitting upright squarely on the seat, legs bent against the pedals or footrest. Your hands are on the handlebar, elbows bent, just in front of your body and over your thighs. To begin to row, extend your arms straight forward, bringing your torso forward from the hips and pulling as far forward as comfortable. If you were in a boat, this would be the *catch* position of the stroke, getting ready to pull or drive the oars through the water (see figure 5.6). Your knees should stay close together so that they come up either under your armpits or in front of your chest. You then simultaneously push your legs and swing your torso back, keeping your arms straight. Only when your legs are fully extended do you begin to pull in with your arms, at the same time finishing the swing of your upper body to a vertical position. Your elbows should be hanging down in a relaxed position, passing closely by your torso as you finish the stroke, or pull (see figure 5.7). You recover by straightening your arms to the start position. As you stop rolling on the seat, you then begin pushing off for the next drive. Keep a relaxed grip on the handles and be sure to sit in the middle of the seat and avoid twisting back and forth. Sound complicated? It is actually easier than it sounds.

Want to work harder? Just by increasing the resistance or the speed of your stroke, you can offer a substantial challenge to your body. For gains in aerobic fitness, you will want to set the resistance at a lower level to work longer while toning your muscles. If you set the resistance levels too high, you will begin to approach the *anaerobic stage* (working without oxygen), and your muscles will get a harder workout. Our goal here is to improve cardiovascular fitness, so working at a lower resistance level will be your best choice.

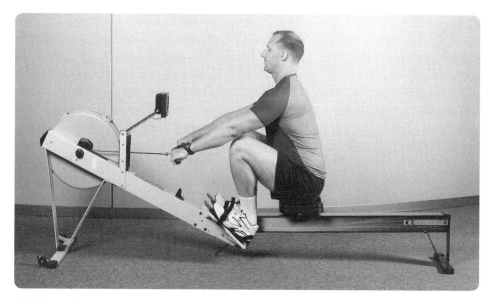

FIGURE 5.6   The catch position.

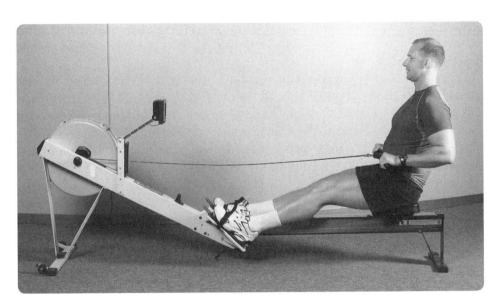

FIGURE 5.7 Position at the end of the stroke.

Posture is important in rowing. It is important to sit as tall as possible and support your low back with your abs. Keeping the abs in will also prevent you from overarching your low back during the end of the stroke as well as help you maintain an erect posture. Make sure you keep your arms close to the sides of your body and squeeze between your shoulder blades as you row back to maximize the work of your upper back. Footwear is recommended; however, all that is necessary are comfortable recreational shoes to protect your feet from the mechanics and track of the machine.

Rowing is a great cardiovascular exercise for increasing endurance and strength through the upper body and the lower body simultaneously. Yet once you are in the rhythm of the movement, it can be a peaceful, stress-reducing way to exercise because it incorporates both the body and, as you concentrate on the movement pattern, the mind.

Jumping Rope

Want to get in touch with your youth again? Do you remember days when you couldn't wait to get outside and get to the playground to play hopscotch, play on the jungle gym, and jump rope? Well, you might have outgrown the hopscotch and jungle gym, but jumping rope is still a form of activity that can bring you a multitude of benefits. It is a fun, energetic way to exercise and allows you to discover your youth again. Jumping rope has many benefits, primarily conditioning your heart and lungs; however, it can increase body awareness and develop better hand and foot coordination. Some of the other benefits of jumping rope are enhanced speed, muscular strength, and endurance; preventing osteoporosis;

and increasing balance and agility. Best of all, jumping rope is an inexpensive activity that is easy to start because the only equipment you need is a jump rope and comfortable shoes.

Jump ropes have changed over the years since we were young. Today they are made from a variety of materials and feature grip handles. Some are weighted or have heavy handles, which can be cumbersome; they are not recommended for aerobic training because they can add stress to the shoulder joints. Choose a lightweight rope with foam grips because they will not slip if your palms become sweaty. They are available in various lengths. To choose the right length for you, stand on the middle of the rope and bring both handles up to your chest. The handles should reach about chest height. The best shoes for jumping rope are cross-trainers or aerobic shoes. Look for good cushioning in the ball of the foot, where you land. Jumping rope is an impact activity, and the cushioning will help you absorb the shock of jumping up and down. A reinforced toe will protect your toes from the rope, and lateral support will give the side-to-side support you need when you land.

The muscles of the lower body, the quadriceps, hamstrings, gluteals, gastrocnemius, and anterior tibialis work to pump the blood through the body to elicit the cardiorespiratory response required to increase your heart rate. The stabilizing muscles of the torso have to work hard to keep your body erect as you jump up and down. When jumping rope, focus on engaging the abdominal and back extensor muscles throughout the workout. Your shoulders should be down and away from your ears to avoid them hunching up toward your ears as the rope travels overhead. Don't grip the handles too tightly—hold them near the ends closest to the rope. Keep your shoulders relaxed and your elbows close to your body. Turn the rope from your wrist and aim to keep a smooth arc in the rope as it passes over your head. When you start to jump, make sure the rope touches the floor slightly. Jump low to the ground to minimize impact and remain in a tall, vertical position. Make sure you bend your knees each time you land. This will help in absorbing shock. See figure 5.8, *a* and *b*, for proper jumping and landing techniques.

The different kinds of jumps and techniques range from easy to extremely challenging. Following are some techniques that range from low to higher intensity. Some of these will be used in the workouts found in later sections of our book.

Low-Intensity Jumping Techniques

Double-foot jump: Both feet take off from the ground and land together.

Alternate-foot jump: In this skipping technique, both feet are alternated up and down while the rope makes its revolution.

Moderate-Intensity Jumping Techniques

Alternate-foot jump: As described in the low-intensity section; this technique can be of low or moderate intensity depending on how fast it's performed.

Running step: A slight jog is incorporated while jumping or skipping over the rope. A slightly faster pace increases the intensity.

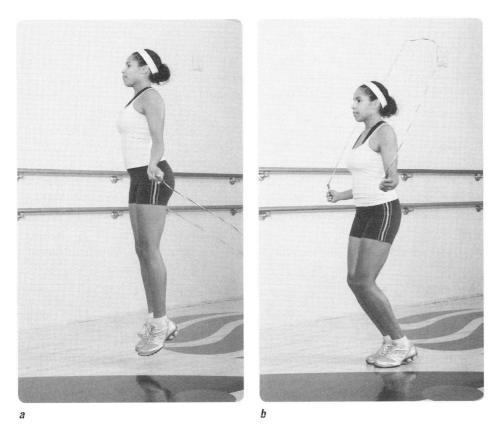

a   *b*

FIGURE 5.8   Proper jumping rope posture: *(a)* jumping; *(b)* landing.

High-Intensity Jumping Techniques

Cross step: While in the air during the jump phase, cross the lower legs slightly and land with legs crossed.

Side to side: Alternate landing areas from left to right. Be careful to pay attention to where the rope might go in this pattern.

In no time you will begin to see a noticeable improvement in your endurance level from jumping rope. It is a great cross-training activity that will certainly add variety to your morning cardio workouts, and who knows—you might just feel like a kid again!

Swimming

There is no question, swimming is great exercise; it is a lifetime sport that benefits the body and the whole person. In addition to increasing your cardiovascular endurance, you also gain muscular strength as you pull your body through the resistance of the water. This resistance allows you to build strength in your limbs and core with every stroke. Swimming is not always convenient (unless you have a pool in your backyard), but the lifetime benefits are worth the effort it takes to get to a pool. And because it is a nonimpact activity (for the most part, your body is supported by the water), it makes for a wonderful addition to your morning cardio workouts. In addition to being nonimpact, swimming also helps improve balance and agility.

Swimming is a great way to burn calories. It burns calories at a rate of three calories a mile per pound of body weight. If you weight 150 pounds (56 kilograms) and it takes you 30 minutes to swim one mile (1.6 kilometers), then you will be using about 900 calories in one hour. That is a fairly quick pace, but it gives you an idea of how effective swimming is at burning calories! The efficiency of your stroke technique determines how many calories you are burning. The more efficient your stroke is, the fewer calories you'll burn. When you are just learning to swim, you use a substantial amount of energy through the mechanics of the learning process. Once you have gained proficiency, however, your stroke will be more efficient. At that point you can increase your speed. Doing so will increase your calorie expenditure.

Don't be fooled by the lower heart rate response in swimming. Your heart rate is lower in the water because water helps cool the body. Also, the physiological response to working out in a horizontal position in buoyant water decreases the heart rate because the body doesn't have to fight against gravity. Because of this, you can exercise your body harder but with less fatigue. The lower heart rate during swimming doesn't mean you are working any less.

Almost every muscle in your body is used in swimming; however, the primary muscles used are the gluteals, hamstrings, and quadriceps as a result of kicking through the water. The upper-body muscles used in swimming include the deltoids (shoulder muscles), latissimus dorsi (back muscles), trapezius, and rhomboids (mid- and upper-back muscles), as well as the biceps and triceps. In some strokes (e.g., the butterfly), the rotator muscles are involved, allowing the shoulders and arms to get a complete workout in all three planes of the body. The abdominal and back extensor muscles stabilize the trunk to maintain the efficiency of the stroke.

Learning how to swim is important because it increases your efficiency in the water as well as your comfort level for other recreational activities such as boating, water skiing, and snorkeling. It is also an enjoyable form of exercise that you can share with the whole family; kids especially like to swim. Following are some basic guidelines for swimming:

- **Maintain a horizontal position using as little energy as possible to displace the most water to the rear.** If your feet are dangling, you are effectively trying to shove a body twice the thickness of yours through the water.

- **Keep your stroke or kick narrow.** You want to push the least surface of yourself forward by occupying the smallest amount of space. Think: Horizontal body, shallow pull, narrow kick.

- **Keep your elbow high at the start so you can pull with your whole arm and not just your upper arm.** Closed fingers are more efficient than wide open fingers, which make a larger surface than closed fingers.

- **Take your time.** The best swimmers tend to take fewer strokes. Concentrate on maintaining a steady pull without losing your attention and letting the water slip by.
- **Relax.** Remember the phrase, If you don't need it, don't use it. You don't need neck muscles to swim, so keep your neck relaxed.
- **Think.** Keep your attention in the moment.

There are a number of swimming strokes and techniques, including the freestyle crawl, the breaststroke, the backstroke, and the butterfly. All are effective styles of swimming, with the freestyle crawl being the most popular. Good mechanics of each stroke are essential in maximizing your efficiency in the water. Following is a review of a few strokes typically used in lap swimming.

- **Freestyle crawl.** You begin this stroke with a push off the wall, straight and narrow. Kick your legs narrowly using your hips to flop your feet. Allow the water to bend your knees slightly. Your arms are straight in front of you, and your hands are flat. Leave the area from your shoulder to your elbow on the surface while your hand drops down until it's below your elbow. Start pulling with your whole arm. Sense what you are doing, trying to feel the pressure of the water along your whole arm, not just your hand. Your arm now looks like a boomerang as you switch from pull to push and increase the pressure. When you think you have completed the push, go another 6 inches (15 centimeters) forcefully. Let the momentum take your elbow out of the water and let your hand dangle behind (see figure 5.9). Your shoulder swings your arm effortlessly all the way straight in front of you. Let the other arm begin its cycle when you are at least halfway through the recovery of the first arm. You will want to breathe in the trough your head makes, so you won't need to lift your head at all. Keep your spine straight as your torso rotates with each stroke, but hold your head steady.

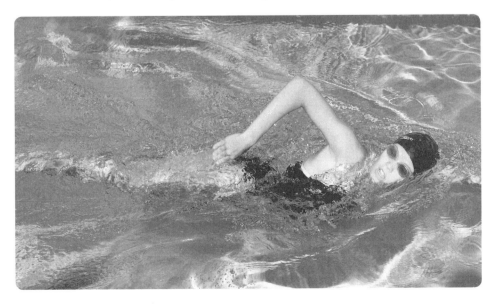

FIGURE 5.9   The freestyle crawl.

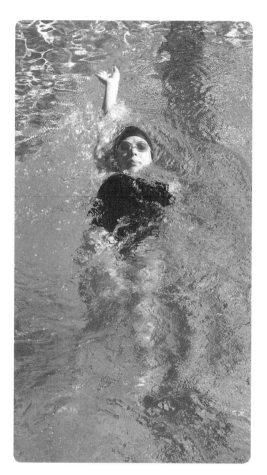

FIGURE 5.10   The backstroke.

• **Backstroke.** Submerged and facing up, push off the wall with your feet. When you surface for your first breath, begin the stroke by lifting one arm out of the water with the thumb facing up. This arm follows a semicircular pattern up and over your shoulders, and the palm rotates outward so that the small finger reenters the water first. As one arm enters the water, the other arm lifts out and follows its own semicircular pattern. Your arms should be 180 degrees from one another during the backstroke. In our backstroke technique, the body roll is more pronounced than in the freestyle technique. When your hand passes your hip, initiate rotation with the hips and roll your body to its side. With your body on its side, you can more easily bend at the elbow, which aids in pulling the arm out of the water. Also with this type of roll, you won't have to reach behind your back to get your arm and hand back into the water. Your body will be on its side, so you are stroking more comfortably because each arm will naturally be in the correct position. Use an alternating leg kick for the backstroke, bending the knee slightly before making a swift upward kick. See figure 5.10 for correct backstroke form.

• **Breaststroke.** Believe it or not, the breaststroke is the most technically demanding swim technique of all. Timing is everything. Your arms and legs are in a streamlined position, as in the freestyle crawl, and they return to that position momentarily on every stroke. As in the freestyle crawl, your elbows stay up as your forearms sweep out and around the body as if inside a big salad bowl, your upper arms snapping together when your hands are coming in under your body, at the bottom of the imagined salad bowl. As your hands, close together, extend forward to their beginning position, your knees bend to bring your feet very close to your butt and pointed out (see figure 5.11). While still extending your arms, your legs imitate your arm stroke, circling out and around and snapping back and together. Hold the glide position for a second. Breathing takes place when your arms, snapping together under your chin, push water up, raising your chin. Your head goes back down as your arms go forward. More than any other stroke, the breaststroke must be watched and imitated.

Swimming is considered a sport with a low risk of injury. Nevertheless, it carries some risks, including the following:

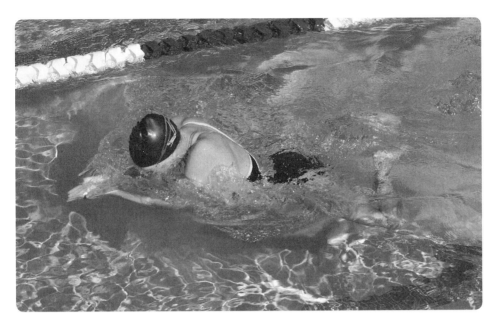

FIGURE 5.11   The breaststroke.

- Exposure to chemicals (chlorine in the eyes or chlorine inhalation).
- Overuse injuries: Competitive butterfly stroke swimmers can develop some back pain and shoulder pain from long bouts of training. Breaststroke swimmers can develop knee pain. Freestyle crawl swimmers may develop *swimmer's shoulder*—a form of tendinitis.
- Diving into a submerged object or the bottom of a pool.
- Exhaustion or unconsciousness.
- Drowning, arising from adverse conditions overwhelming the swimmer or causing water inhalation.

Taking the proper precautions can help avoid many, if not all, of the preceding situations. We recommend that you swim in an area supervised by lifeguards. The use of goggles and nose plugs may help you adjust to the elements of water.

You have a couple of options for your swimming workouts: leisure swimming and lap swimming. Perhaps you prefer a nonstructured type of workout in which you work out at your own pace. If so, then leisure swimming might be the choice for you. Leisure swimming allows you to choose a style that works best for you, maybe even using a variety of strokes, to help you reach your fitness goals. You make it as hard or as easy as you wish. As long as you swim continuously, you will get a complete aerobic workout. This method is typically used for maintenance of your fitness level rather than increasing your level because you are working at a low to moderate intensity level. You shouldn't feel exhausted or completely breathless during a leisure swim. Maintain a rhythmic and steady pace to ensure the aerobic benefit of the workout.

When you don't feel quite up to pushing yourself yet you want to get a cardio-vascular workout, the leisure swim may be the choice for you. There are other psychological benefits to this style of swimming—if you allow them to occur. While working at a low or moderate pace, you can relax and swim with less effort. In this way you can let your mind wander, focusing on nothing but the rhythm of your stroke. This form of meditation can help you gain a feeling of well-being, and you will leave your water session refreshed and ready to go on with the rest of your day. The backstroke might be a good choice because it allows you to breathe whenever and however you want, although you will probably form a pattern and stick with it without even realizing it. The breaststroke and freestyle crawl would also be good choices for this type of swimming because both require that the arms and legs be in a streamlined position.

Leisure swimming will allow you to burn enough calories to enjoy a guilt-free breakfast as well as dedicating time to yourself to help you stay in the moment.

If structure is more your cup of tea, then lap swimming may be the style for you. Lap swimming entails using different strokes such as the freestyle crawl, breaststroke, backstroke, or butterfly to get across the pool in the most efficient way possible. It is usually performed in continuous motion at a higher intensity level than that of leisure swimming. Typically, you choose a style of swimming that suits you and perform that style throughout a lap. At the completion of the lap, you execute a flip turn with a push off the wall to propel you into the next lap while keeping the rhythm and pace of the stroke. Sometimes the flip turn will signal the initiation of another stroke. This technique allows you to keep your heart rate elevated in an effort to maintain or increase your cardiovascular response.

Most facilities with indoor pools hold lanes open for lap swimming in the early mornings, making this a convenient way to get in your morning cardio workout. Often they have lanes marked for both slower and faster swimmers. If you find that you are consistently getting passed or are slowing other swimmers down, you might want to move to a slower lane so as not to disrupt other swimmers' workouts. On the contrary, if you are a faster swimmer and are consistently pass-ing others, you should move to the fast lane or just along the outside of the lane to keep the lanes moving well.

Swimming has benefited many over the years and offers all the components to help you achieve your fitness goals. It meets the criteria for attaining gains in cardiovascular fitness, muscular strength, and endurance, and above all else, it makes you feel great! It is a refreshing, effective and wonderful way to begin your day. Swim on!

Pool Walking

If you have ever tried to run or walk quickly to get out of a pool, then you have had the opportunity to experience the difficulty of moving fast in water. This is the premise behind pool walking, an effective, easy-to-learn water activity that requires absolutely no swimming skills! This form of exercise is performed in waist- to shoulder-deep water.

Pool walking combines the toning of weight training, the cardiovascular benefits of aerobics, and the enhanced flexibility gained through yoga—all in about 30 minutes per day! Water is a natural and instantly adjustable weight training machine, providing resistance in all directions to tone and strengthen the muscles. Because of this, pool walking promotes balance in muscular development in addition to the cardiovascular benefits you achieve. The same muscles used in walking on land, the lower leg muscles—gluteals, quadriceps, hamstrings, gastrocnemius, anterior tibialis, and ankle muscles—are all used in the water as well. Water workouts effectively burn fat and strengthen the abdominal muscles without doing a single sit-up! This is the result of your body's stabilizing itself while maintaining balance as it reacts to the buoyancy of the water surrounding you. The movements are low impact and joint friendly, helping to prevent injuries as well as heal them. Choose this type of workout when looking to avoid jarring and high-impact activities, when you want to add a little variety to your cross-training routine, or when you want to perform a cardiovascular routine that will also enhance leg strength.

Footwear is suggested for pool walking and pool running. Pool bottoms can be slippery, especially the lane markers painted on the bottom of the pool. In addition, when you jump or run in the water, you are adding impact to your activity. Although the impact is less because of the cushioning effect of the water, there is still impact. A good aqua shoe with cushioning and lateral support will help protect your limbs, back, and knees from the potential shock of impact. Aqua shoes are available at sporting goods outlets. They are lightweight and dry quickly. These shoes are meant to be worn without socks, so be sure to try them on without socks before buying.

In water, resistance determines your intensity. You are in charge! You choose the intensity level by incorporating speed, force, or surface area The larger the surface area presented against the water is, the greater the resistance is. Adding arm movements under the water will add to the challenge because the arms have to work to propel you through the water. Also, by increasing your speed, you increase the intensity of the workout. The higher the water level is, the more challenging the workout will be. Start pool walking in waist-deep water and increase to chest level for maximum benefit.

Before your pool walking workout, it is important to warm up first by walking slowly for the first five minutes. Once you begin your workout, start at one end of the pool or lap lane and walk at a moderate, comfortable pace across the pool to the other side and back. You can vary your workout and increase the intensity by adding arm and leg movements. Extend your arms out to the side, keeping them underwater. With palms facing forward, bring your arms toward each other with fingers closed and cross them in front of you, then turn your palms back and push them back. Swoop both arms from side to side, alternating using both arms and using individual arms. Vary your leg movements—create a letter V, stepping "out, out, in, in" as you walk across the pool. Step forward and lift one knee toward your chest, repeating with the other leg. Follow your workout with a cool-down in the water for about five minutes with gentle relaxing moves to bring your heart rate back to where it was when you started.

Pool Running

Perhaps you need a break from the impact of day-to-day fitness activities. Maybe you've been hurt and need a nonimpact way of keeping fit. Or perhaps you want a gentle, refreshing, yet effective way to work out. Pool running, whether in shallow or deep water, can do the trick! It is an effective aerobic workout, certainly gets your heart rate up, pumps your muscles, and will leave you feeling as though you've had a full-body massage. What a wonderful way to start your day!

Pool running is a wonderful alternative to running on land. It is easier on the joints, increases range of motion, rehabilitates injuries, and builds sport-specific strength—making running on land easier and more fluid. Athletic trainers and coaches are now incorporating shallow- and deep-water running into their athletes' training because they have found that the training benefits achieved in the water cross over to the demands of their sports on land. It is also a good exercise if you are pregnant because the water keeps your temperature fairly even, and it eliminates the stress on your body and joints by providing cushioning and support.

For effective pool running, make sure you have proper form. Keep your abdominal muscles contracted to support your back, and avoid leaning forward from the waist. As you run, raise your knees to about hip height, then push down and slightly backward with your foot. Bend your arms at a 90-degree angle and swing them from your shoulders. Allow your fingers to come just below the surface of the water in front of you, and to your hips at your side in the backward swing. To increase intensity, try to run harder by moving your arms and legs faster. The faster you run, or push, the harder the workout will be because of the resistance of the water against the push.

In shallow-water running, you are in water from waist to chest deep and your feet are in contact with the pool bottom, as in pool walking. In deep-water running, you are suspended vertically in the water by wearing a flotation belt. It's as though you are running in midair!

• **Shallow-water running.** Shallow-water running is performed in water from waist-deep to shoulder-deep levels. The deeper the water is, the more intense the workout is because more body parts are submerged. Because your feet are in contact with the bottom of the pool as in pool walking, this an impact activity (i.e., you rebound from one foot to another as you do when running on land). The difference is that the buoyancy and properties of the water cushion the landing to absorb the impact, thereby reducing the amount of shock to the legs and back. For this reason, pool running is a great choice for runners looking to take a break from the jarring impact of their daily running. Footwear is recommended for this activity. As with pool walking, choose a shoe that is flexible and has cushioning. Most aqua shoes are lightweight and dry quickly. Remember—no socks!

For variety you can run across the pool from one wall to the other or stay in place and focus on lifting your knees. It is important to move your arms as well to increase your heart rate. Exaggerate the arm movements to get the most out of your workout by pushing and pulling the water (see figure 5.12). Interval training can be incorporated into pool running. By working harder in intervals, followed by an active recovery of working at your normal training pace, you can train your system to work at higher intensities for longer periods of time. Shallow-water running allows you to train with less impact to your joints, which might allow you to train longer than you would be able to on land. For this reason, shallow-water running is a good choice for those looking to increase the duration of their running workouts with less strain to the body. For a workout that takes the impact completely out of the picture and presents an entirely new dimension to running, deep-water running is worth a try.

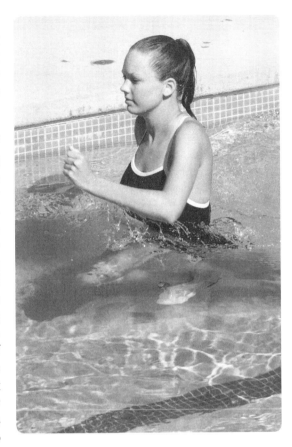

FIGURE 5.12   Correct shallow-water running form.

• **Deep-water running.** Let's get vertical! Deep-water running, in which you are suspended vertically in water wearing a floatation belt, is a perfect cross-training activity. Just by participating in deep-water running, you are helping yourself prevent injury! And if you are already injured (we hope not, but let's face it, it does occasionally happen to the best of us), deep-water running is perfect for keeping your fitness up while your injury heals. Be aware that in the pool your heart rate will be 10 to 15 beats less than it is on land. This is due to the physiological response of the heart when the body is submerged in water. This doesn't mean you are working any less; in fact, your muscles will have to work harder in water than they do on land!

In deep-water running, you wear a flotation belt (available at most swimming specialty stores) around your waist or torso. The belt holds you vertical in the water without your feet touching the pool bottom. This is the difference between shallow-water running and deep-water running. Your head and the tops of your shoulders are out of the water. You will need to be in a pool anywhere from 5 to 6 feet (152 to 183 centimeters) in depth, depending on how tall you are. Some people deep-water run without a belt; however, a belt will allow you to stay tall

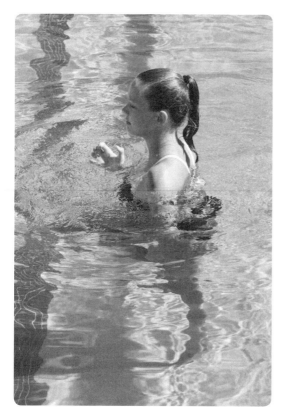

FIGURE 5.13   Correct deep-water running form.

and not lean forward from your back, helping you stay focused on getting your heart rate up rather than on staying afloat or upright. Also, you can use your belt as a tether to tie yourself to the side of the pool so you can work harder by running against the tether.

The goal of deep-water running is to stay in one place by pushing and pulling the water at the same time. The key is balance and core strength. Keep yourself as upright as possible, with your abs held in tight, and your head looking straight ahead (see figure 5.13). Make sure you don't bend forward from the waist and stick out your butt. Push your feet up and down to a 90-degree angle rather than moving them in a cycling motion. Your arms stay as close to your body as possible with a 90-degree bend in the elbow and palms facing the body with thumbs up. To increase the intensity, you can rotate your palms down toward the water, which increases the surface area. You can do interval training drills by running a minute fast and a minute slow, alternating for as long as you want, which is similar to the interval drill in shallow-water running, or you can just re-create the same workouts you do on land.

Water exercise in the form of running is a great way to cross-train and save your legs! You will be saving some of the miles in your legs for another day. Some athletes shrug and shy away from water exercise, claiming they don't like the water. But my theory is, you don't know until you try it! Not only is it effective, but it is also great on hot days. On cold winter days, the warm pool is a wonderful retreat. The best part is that water running will protect and save your joints and will allow you to keep those morning cardio workouts going for years to come.

6

Group Exercise

It's been said that there's strength in numbers, and that adage can apply to working out in groups. The group fitness classes in clubs around the world today are more exciting and varied than ever before. The purpose of this chapter is to give you some options to explore for your morning cardio workout in the group fitness arena.

Group Exercise Terminology

In the 1970s, when the concept of movement classes was new, *aerobics* was a generic term used to describe just about any type of movement class. The term today has been replaced by more specific names of group movement classes. Because the word *aerobics* really refers to any activity involving breathing (*aerobics* itself means "in the presence of oxygen"), class names now more aptly refer to the activities involved, such as "Cardio Dance" and "Low-Impact Combinations."

Later on in this chapter, we will discuss *circuit* and *interval* classes, but these words can refer to techniques as well. Any of the classes discussed in this chapter that adapt a circuit technique format will consist of several small stations of activity. A dance circuit class, for example, could have periods of tango, meringue, and jazz. Any class that adopts an interval format will consist of a manipulation

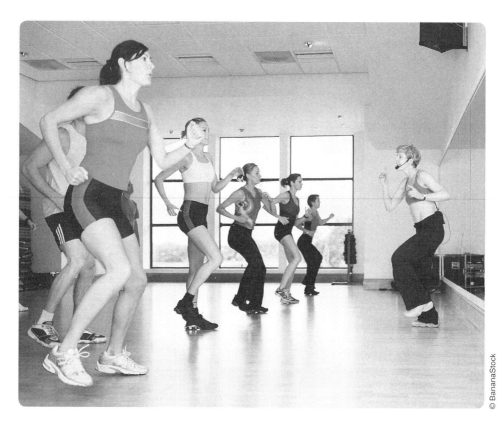

© BananaStock

Adding variety to your routine, group classes will help you remain interested in exercising and committed to your morning workouts.

of intensity in which some periods of the class are more intense than others. In a cycle interval class, for example, some periods of the class will be at a higher intensity than others.

Types of Group Exercise Classes

Working out in small or large groups can enhance motivation, increase adherence to an exercise program, encourage healthy competition, and create a sense of camaraderie, among other things. Look for the types of classes discussed in this chapter at your local gym or fitness club. You may want to learn about different clubs in your area to see which offers as many of the options here as possible. In group fitness, remember that your body becomes efficient the more you take the same types of classes over time, so results can diminish if you attend the same class for months. To make improvements, follow our suggestions endorsing change. Finally, remember that instructors have different teaching styles. Find a style that matches what you find attractive and motivating—for your brain, body, and breath—in your morning cardio workouts. Although some may find the intricate choreography of a difficult step class appealing at 5:00 a.m., you may not. Finally, although the norm is still a range of classes lasting 60 minutes, both shorter classes ("express-style" 30- and 45-minute classes) and longer classes (90-minute yoga classes) are popping up as clubs continue to adapt to changing consumer schedules and needs.

- **High-impact workouts.** The purpose of high-impact cardiovascular workouts is to tax the heart and musculoskeletal system by having the body jump against the earth's surface many times in the course of the workout. This improves not only cardiovascular fitness, but bone density as well (American Council on Exercise 2004; Gladwin 2003). In the fitness world, *high impact* often is defined as when both feet simultaneously leave the floor at certain moments. Such classes have names such as "Hi-Impact," "Hi Cardio Dance," and "Fat Burner." High-impact training classes should occur at a cadence below 155 beats per minute to maximize safety and minimize risk of injury (American Council on Exercise 2004; Gladwin 2003). To *maintain* your fitness level, try to attend three to five of such 60-minute classes per week. To vary the muscles you use and the way your heart is taxed, attend different types of classes, such as those that emphasize the lower body (jump rope classes, modern dancing, jazz, cardio boot camp) and those that emphasize the upper body (boxing, choreography). To *improve* your fitness level during high-impact cardiovascular workouts, change the class type every time you work out, taking between four and six classes per week. Furthermore, try taking interval classes (with peaks of high intensity interspersed with a bit lower intensity or active recovery) instead of maintenance classes. An interval class includes bouts of intense periods of cardiovascular work interspersed with bouts of less intense periods, called active recovery. Your fitness level improves because you train your heart to react to immediate, increased cardiovascular demands. Then, instead of returning to a state of rest, the heart must recover while still being taxed, although to a lesser degree. Interval training is a science unto itself, and we discuss more interval ideas throughout this book.

- **Low-impact workouts.** We define low-impact cardiovascular exercise as that in which at least one foot remains in contact with the floor at all times. The purpose is the same as high-impact cardiovascular exercise, without the jumping action; it is less jarring to joints and appeals to a wide population. Contrary to some opinions, low-impact exercise is *not* less intense than high-impact exercise; indeed, it can be even more so. For example, it is possible to jog or jump rope in place (an example of high impact because both feet leave the floor simultaneously) at a very low intensity so that the feet don't rise off the floor very high. Conversely, a low-impact move can be much more intense, such as a low-impact jumping jack in which you shift your weight from one side to the other, as if stepping out in a side squat, simultaneously raising the arms overhead. Another example of an intense cardiovascular move that is extremely low impact would be squatting so low you touch the floor with your palms, jumping your legs out behind you, jumping your legs back again between your hands to the deep squat, and then standing up. Bone density benefits also occur in low-impact activities, although to a slightly lesser degree because the impact of bones against the floor surfaces is less. Low-impact exercise classes may have names such as, "Low Impact," "Low Impact, High Energy," or "Light and Low." Low-impact training classes should occur at a cadence below 140 beats per minute to maximize safety and minimize risk of injury. To *maintain* your fitness level in these types of classes, try to attend four to six of such 60-minute classes per week. To *improve* your cardiovascular fitness level, think about interspersing one high-impact class between every two low-impact classes to create change and surprise for the musculoskeletal and cardiovascular systems. In order to *improve* your fitness level for low-impact cardiovascular workouts try to take between five to six classes per week, being sure to challenge your intensity appropriately so you feel that you are working out "very hard." You also may wish to take a different type of low-impact cardiovascular exercise class from elsewhere in this chapter.

• **Mixed-impact workouts.** Mixed-impact cardiovascular classes are the most popular today because they offer an exciting combination of the two modalities. Participants of all levels can attend classes and choose to make almost any movement high impact or low impact; thus, one class can cater to many people. To *maintain* your fitness level in these types of classes, try to attend four to six of such 60-minute classes per week. To *improve* your cardiovascular fitness level, think about taking mixed-impact classes that will each challenge your muscles in a different way—such as taking a boxing class on one day and a dance class on another. In order to *improve* your fitness level for mixed-impact cardiovascular workouts try to take between four to six classes per week.

• **Step training.** Step training involves stepping (and sometimes jumping, hopping, and leaping) up and down from a 4- to 10-inch (10- to 25-centimeter) platform. The purpose of step training is to tax the heart while challenging the legs and gluteal muscles. Typical classes on group exercise schedules are called "Step," "Boot Camp Step" (emphasizing more athletic-type drills without complex choreography), "Cardio Step," and "Step Dance" (emphasizing more complex choreography to experienced steppers). Step training classes should occur at a cadence below 130 beats per minute to maximize safety and minimize risk of injury (Miller 1994). To *maintain* your fitness level in these types of classes, try to attend three or four such 60-minute classes per week. To *improve* your cardiovascular fitness level, think about attending different types of step classes. Some step classes will maintain your heart rate at a steady state of training, whereas others (such as those that include more athletic types of drills) will train your cardiovascular system in a more interval-type way. Part of step training's popularity stems from its use of standardized moves and cueing; steppers can attend a step class anywhere in the world and know that the instructors will be drawing from the same set of moves. Having a repertoire of specific moves can also be a comforting alternative for someone who finds the potentially unlimited number of moves used in general dance classes to be overwhelming.

• **Indoor cycling.** Indoor cycling training remains one of the most popular morning cardio workouts. The reason may be that these cycling classes are usually shorter than other classes (45 rather than 60 minutes), and they are often the first class of the day on group fitness schedules. The purpose of indoor group cycling is to train the heart primarily via interval or steady state training, with an increase in leg and gluteal strength as a by-product. A great advantage of adding indoor cycling to your morning cardio workouts is that you get to experience a simulated outdoor activity anytime, regardless of your geographic location and outside weather. Typical classes on group exercise schedules are called "Interval Cycle" (emphasizing an interval ride), and "Recover Ride" (emphasizing steady state training). For overall safety, cycling training classes should involve revolutions per minute that remain between 80 and 110 (Reebok University 1980). To *maintain* your fitness level for these types of classes, attend rides that include steady state training for most of the class time (an indication would be music that does not vary between slow and fast). These types of classes are typically less common than interval rides, however. To *improve* your cardiovascular fitness, attend the more traditional type of cycling class that intersperses higher-intensity activities with lower-intensity activities; this is called interval training. Most classes recommend rating of perceived intensity of between 7 and 9 for the bulk of the cycle ride. (See pages 92 and 93 for information on rate of perceived intensity.) A more detailed description of interval training concludes this chapter.

- **Shallow- and deep-water training.** Water training (also called "aquatic training") means working in water either with the feet touching the pool or ocean bottom (*shallow-water training*) or with the body suspended in a vertical position with a special flotation belt (*deep-water training*). The purpose of water training is to tax the heart and musculoskeletal systems in a more challenging way than on land. Other benefits include a decreased jarring impact to the bones and spine, less awareness of intensity through sweating, increased enjoyment through group dynamics, a constant changing of equipment because of the plethora of aquatic aids available, and the manipulation of the following principles unique to water training: drag, acceleration, and buoyancy (Kravitz and Mayo 1997).

Drag refers to the displacement of water molecules against a moving object, which means that the larger the surface area of an object moving through the water is, the more force that object has to generate to accomplish that movement. A fascinating fact about drag is that water has 12 times the drag of air. Just walking through water is 12 times harder than walking through air so you need to work 12 times harder in the water than on land! *Acceleration* refers to the speed of movement achieved from touching other molecules. This can refer to the bottom and sides of the pool or to the water itself. Finally, buoyancy refers to the ability of an object to move in opposition to being submerged and, consequently, float.

Typical aquatic classes listed on group-exercise schedules are called "Aquatic Fitness," "Water Walking/Jogging," "Aqua Circuit," "Liquid Strength," and so on. Because some classes emphasize strength while others emphasize cardiovascular endurance, there is no ideal recommendation of beats per minute for all classes. To *maintain* your fitness level for these types of classes, try to attend between three and five aquatic classes per week that emphasize cardiovascular endurance over strength. To *improve* your cardiovascular fitness, try to attend between four and six aquatic classes per week. These classes should vary in depth (shallow or deep), equipment used, and, most importantly, intensity.

If you find that you have reached a point at which you notice no further changes or improvements in your fitness level, you may have reached what is referred to as a fitness plateau. The solution when reaching a plateau is to shake up the exercise routine with new muscular stimuli via new exercises. The aquatic environment is often the most overlooked solution to getting over a fitness plateau. Because water offers more resistance than air, just taking a walking routine you are currently doing into the water will guarantee more caloric expenditure, improved cardiovascular benefits, and an entirely new facet to fitness enjoyment.

• **Fusion formats.** Fusion formats are quickly becoming popular as more fitness enthusiasts realize the benefits of getting away from a plateau and begin to change their routines with interval and circuit formats. A fusion workout, sometimes referred to as a hybrid workout, is one that puts together modalities that normally wouldn't occur in the same type of class. The purpose of a fusion class is to give you more benefits than you would experience if you had to choose just one modality. Another purpose is to help the busy exerciser of today experience more benefits in less time. To be sure, some fusion formats emphasize strength (such as weightlifting and Pilates) and flexibility (such as tai chi and yoga), but we emphasize here those that fuse cardiovascular benefits. Examples of such fusion formats appearing on group exercise classes are "Step and Hi-Lo Cardio," "Cycling and BOSU Balance Trainer Fusion" (BOSU stands for "**BO**th **S**ides **U**tilized," in which half of a stability ball is attached to a flat platform and placed on the floor), and "Water Cardio Fusion: Deep and Shallow." Because this trend is so new, fusion may just be the type of group workout you have not yet discovered that will tax your cardiovascular system with a plethora of stimuli as you maximize results in the shortest amount of time possible!

• **Interval training.** Interval training means training the heart through a manipulation of intensity levels. This can refer either to a technique used during a class or to a class itself. During interval training, you tax your heart and then let it recover while you continue to work at a less intense level. Traditionally, the objective has been to raise the work level to that intensity, sustain it there, and transition to a different intensity level. In interval training formats, however, you raise your work level and then from that state occasionally go higher to an anaerobic state (workout without oxygen, almost breathless). You then return to the original level which is *not* rest, but the previous aerobic state. This state is called active recovery, and the exercise intensity is low enough to facilitate the removal of lactate, a by-product of one of the systems that creates energy for your body.

The great advantage to interval training is that more work is done in the same amount of time as in a traditional class, offering such benefits as more caloric expenditure, more cardiovascular training, and more $\dot{V}O_2$max training. $\dot{V}O_2$max *training* refers to the capacity of the lungs to use air; the more fit you are, the higher your $\dot{V}O_2$max is. Research shows that to burn more calories, you need to work out at a higher intensity (Kravitz 1994; McArdle, Katch, and Katch 1998). You increase your fitness level because after you work really hard (between 1 minute and 90 seconds), you don't return to rest but instead just ease up on the intensity, forcing your heart to recover while you are still exercising. To *maintain* your fitness level, you should have your intense work time occur at either the same rate or at a shorter rate than your recovery time. An example might be running (the intense part) for one minute and then running more slowly (the active recovery part) for one or two minutes. To *improve* your fitness level, your work time must exceed your recovery time, so you would run for one minute and walk for less than that (e.g., 30 seconds).

Interval training differs from steady state training. The latter refers to any cardiovascular activity aimed at maintaining your heart rate at a consistent level. If you are deconditioned or new to fitness, steady state training will improve your fitness level. However, if you are an avid exerciser, steady state training will *maintain* your fitness level and you will eventually reach a cardiovascular plateau. To *improve* your fitness level, think about incorporating some interval training into your program to change your routine and make your body work harder via active recovery.

- **Circuit training.** Circuit training relates more to specific exercises than to exercise intensity. The purpose of circuit training is to address different modes of exercises within a relatively short time. A circuit could be aerobic, anaerobic, strength, or a combination of these with designated times for each, called stations. To *maintain* your fitness level, you can choose at least two cardiovascular modalities and vary them equally. For example, you can alternate between walking and running for five-minute segments. Although it's also an interval because of intensity, it's a circuit because you have chosen two different types of cardiovascular exercise. To *improve* your cardiovascular strength and endurance, you can choose several types of cardiovascular exercise and intersperse these with some strength moves that keep your heart rate elevated while increasing muscle mass. For example, you can intersperse running and walking for five minutes with one to three minutes of squatting in place.

In short, one of the most significant ways to improve your cardiovascular strength in your morning cardio workouts is to incorporate interval and circuit training (American Council on Exercise 2003, 2004; Gladwin 2003) Because both interval and circuit training depend on the two factors of intensity and exercise choice, almost any type of workout or class (step, cycle, low-impact cardiovascular training) can incorporate interval or circuit training. These types of training prepare you to handle life's challenges because life's intensity is never constant: Change is certain! Daily activities often involve sudden changes in intensity and duration with little warning (such as driving a car and suddenly hopping out to run into the grocery store). Interval and circuit training can help you handle daily stresses.

part two

Workouts for Every Morning

By now you have all the information you need to get started. You have checked out your options, learned the best way to fuel your body, taken inventory of how your body responds, and familiarized yourself with staying focused and connected with our brain–body–breath concepts. It is now time to learn and understand how to put it all into practice. We have done the work for you. All you have to do is determine your goal for the day or week, choose your activity, choose the intensity level that you feel will best match that goal, determine how much time you want or have to devote today, and carpe diem! Seize your day!

How to Use the Workouts in the Book

The workouts in this part are divided into categories. Do you feel like an easy workout this morning? Then check out the options in the light workout category (chapter 7). These workouts are perfect when you feel the need to work out, but your body is telling you to pull back a bit. They are designed to elevate your heart rate and will allow you to burn calories and maintain your fitness levels while working at an intensity that will minimize stress to your joints. Your brain–body–breath connection can come to life as you get in the rhythm of a light and easier workout.

Are you feeling like a bit of a challenge this morning? Then choose a workout plan from the moderate category (chapter 8). These workouts are designed to help you increase your heart rate response as you put a bit more effort into your workout. Your intensity level will be a bit higher here as you gently push yourself a bit further. Your brain–body–breath connection is important here as you concentrate on how your body responds to the increased intensity levels and make sure you stay true to your form.

Do you need this morning to be the day to push yourself to the limit? Then choose a workout plan from the intense category (chapter 9). If your goal is to increase your fitness levels and see significant changes such as losing weight or training for an event, you will want to incorporate one or two of the intense morning workouts a week to allow you to reach your goal. These workouts are designed to take you a little beyond your normal workout levels, so be sure that you have taken the time to build yourself up by using the light and moderate workouts to get you there. Use your brain–body–breath connection, and listen to your body and how it responds to the increased demands. The human body is an amazing machine, and it was designed to move and respond positively to training. You will be pleasantly surprised to see how your fitness levels improve in only a short time.

Remember to balance your workouts and incorporate recovery workouts (chapter 10) into your weekly routine. Yes, we have also included recovery workouts for you to choose from. You have it all!

Each workout is organized in an easy-to-follow format. We include an introduction to give you a general idea of what your workout is about and what your focus should be. We have divided the workouts into time allotments with intensity level checks during each. Each time frame has some tips to help you through the workouts. For more technique tips, refer to the activity descriptions in chapters 3, 4, and 5. Each workout is complete and includes a cool-down, so you can go from start to finish in the time you have allotted for your workout. Sound easy? It is!

How to Measure Your Intensity

When people find they are not reaching their fitness goals, it is usually because they are not working at an adequate intensity. What makes a workout effective is its intensity. In chapter 5 we discussed the difference between impact and intensity. Impact does not determine your intensity level. Intensity is the amount of effort you put into your workout.

By nature some activities are more intense than others. Some require training to be able to participate at the intensity and impact levels they require. For example, race walking is more intense than fitness walking and requires that you work up to the intensity level. Some people, because of biomechanical limitations, may never be able to reach the intensity level of race walking. The key to success is to choose an activity that you *enjoy* and can physically participate in at the correct intensity level. In this section, instead of listing activities in the order of their intensity, we review how to monitor your intensity by rating your perceived exertion.

Perceived exertion is a method of determining your intensity level based on the way you feel. It reflects the interaction between your mind and your body. Because it matches our philosophy regarding the brain–body–breath connection, it is a perfect fit for morning cardio workouts. The physiological experience is linked to the physiological events that occur in physical exercise. Perceived exertion is a subjective judgment because it incorporates information about how you feel both emotionally and physically. The greater the frequency of your signals—your breathing, your muscle response, etc.—the more intense you will find your perception of exertion to be. Studies show that the exertion scale proves a relationship between your heart rate and the amount of oxygen you are taking in during aerobic exercise.

For the purposes of this book and our workouts, we will use a perceived exertion scale of 1 to 10 (1 being the easiest and 10 being the hardest exertion for any given session). This allows you to evaluate how hard you have worked in any given workout session. One indicates extremely light exertion, such as sitting at rest, where breathing is comfortable and at a normal pace. We typically use three through five to indicate a progressive warm-up pace. At three, movement takes minimal effort and breathing is comfortable; at five, exertion becomes somewhat difficult, and breath and physical exertion become apparent. We typically use seven through nine to indicate moderate to intense effort. At seven, movement is difficult and a heavier breath pattern is apparent; at nine, movement is extremely difficult and a person becomes breathless. Ten indicates maximal exertion.

The underlying theory of perceived exertion is that we each have an optimum training level. Every session we perform should have a preassigned exertion number that correlates to the objectives of the workout. We recommend that sessions be performed in the 5 to 8.5 range, depending on your goal for the morning, to achieve optimal results. But know that you should always listen to your body and work within your limits. There is no right or wrong way to rate your perceived exertion. Just become familiar with the guidelines of the scale and rate yourself based on how hard you feel you are working.

Although there are no right or wrong ratings, it helps to clearly understand the meaning of the descriptions. You want to relate how you feel you are working aerobically as well as how your muscles are responding, particularly your legs.

Listen to your body, focus on your breath, and allow your mind to guide you as you find your path to improved fitness with these early morning workouts. Carpe diem! You are ready to go.

7

Light Workouts

This chapter includes light workouts. They are perfect for those who are just starting to work out, as well as for those looking to complement heavy training days.

Each workout starts with a complete warm-up. Be sure to follow the guidelines listed, as the warm-up specifically prepares you for the rest of the workout to follow.

As you begin your workout, take the time to incorporate a visualization that will help you make the most of the brain–body–breath connection. For example, if you have chosen a rowing workout, close your eyes, breathe deeply, and imagine that you are about to glide across a serene lake on a beautiful, sunny day. Feel the cool breeze on your face as you increase the intensity of your workout, and imagine the wonderful smells of the greenery surrounding the lake's edge. Or, if you have chosen a stair stepper workout, close your eyes, breathe deeply, and imagine you are about to hike up a natural stone trail nestled in the foothills of a mountain range. Envision the beauty of the surrounding land on a warm, sunny day, and imagine the sounds of rushing water drifting toward you from a nearby creek. These visualizations will help make your morning workout an adventure that will leave you empowered, invigorated, and refreshed.

A cool-down is also incorporated into each workout—for recovery workout ideas, please refer to chapter 10.

Lastly, the "RPE" appearing in the second column of the tables throughout the chapter refers to the *rate of perceived exertion*. The section titled "How to Measure Your Intensity" on page 92 provides the guidelines for measuring exertion levels.

20-Minute Light Workouts

Leisure Walking—Flat Terrain

The morning is a beautiful time to walk outside and enjoy the fresh air and the radiant sunrise. Try to use all your senses and pay attention to the birds chirping and the smell of the air around you. For this workout you will want to find a walking path that is fairly flat with no hills. The goal for this workout is to increase cardiovascular endurance.

Minutes	RPE	Instruction
1-5	4	Warm-up: Start out at an easy pace; your arms should sway gently forward and back.
6-8	5	Be aware of rolling through your entire foot from heel to toe.
9-11	5	Keep your abdominal muscles in tight and focus on pulling your navel toward your spine.
12-15	5	Alternately walk on the balls of your feet and on your heels in 30- to 45-second intervals. Keep your arms close to your sides. Avoid swinging your arms across your body.
16-18	5	Focus on swinging your arms forward and back.
19-20	4-5	Cool-down: Focus on your breath to decrease your heart rate.

Fitness Walking—Rolling Hills

Clear your mind of everything that happened yesterday. This morning is a new day. Take the time to center yourself and focus on being in the present moment. Find a marked trail or sidewalk that starts off level and then slopes uphill and downhill multiple times. You want your intensity to increase for about three minutes and then to recover for about three minutes. The goals of this workout are to increase cardiovascular strength and endurance with interval training, empower you with a positive attitude, and help keep you on task for the rest of the day.

Minutes	RPE	Instruction
1-5	4	Warm-up: Start out at an easy pace; your arms should sway gently forward and back.
6-8	5	Continue at the same pace and start pumping your arms faster by your sides.
9-11	7	Here you will be starting up your first hill. Focus on pulling your navel toward your spine and keeping your back straight. Try not to lean forward from your hips.
12-14	5	Recovery time coming down the hill; stay light on your feet.
15-17	7	Hill #2: Increase your pace and pump those arms.
18-20	4-5	Cool-down: Focus on your breath as you come down the hill and feel the calming of your breath as your heart rate quickly lowers.

Road Biking—Flat Terrain

Biking early in the morning is an excellent way to work out. You don't have to worry as much about traffic, and in hot summer months the weather tends to be much cooler. The cool air hitting your face and the fresh morning scents energize you for the rest of the day. For this workout a flat or dirt road or paved bike path with no hills works best. Avoid trails with heavy, loose gravel. County, township, or state parks are great resources for this activity because the paths are designed with safety in mind. The goals of this workout are to increase cardiovascular endurance and build strength in your legs.

Minutes	RPE	Instruction
1-5	4	Warm-up: Maintain even pedal strokes, keeping your feet flat and your ankle joints flexed.
6-18	5	Increase your intensity a bit. Focus on maintaining a stable posture, engaging your abdominal muscles and maintaining strong and stable shoulders with your chest open. Keep a neutral wrist position.
19-20	4-5	Cool-down: Focus on your breath and slow down your pedal stroke.

Treadmill

Treadmills have become one of the most popular pieces of exercise equipment today. The early morning scenes at clubs and exercise facilities validate the popularity of this workout: Almost every treadmill is typically occupied. In addition, many people have treadmills in their homes. This is a great way to jump out of bed and get your cardio workout in before you have to shower and get ready for the rest of your day. Treadmill walking is a low-impact workout that is easy on your joints. This workout is designed for the sole purpose of burning calories. You will not see significant gains in cardiovascular function or capacity, but you will keep the metabolic furnace fired up. Remember, it doesn't *always* have to be super intense to get maximum results—change makes change, and by continually switching intensity and duration, your body will inevitably respond.

Minutes	RPE	Instruction
1-5	4-5	Warm-up: Start at an easy pace; your arms should sway forward and back.
6-8	6.5	Focus on your feet and rolling through your second toe.
9-17	6	Pump your arms, keeping them close to your sides.
18-20	5	Cool-down: Focus on how your body feels by mentally scanning your body from head to toe.

20-Minute Light Workouts

Elliptical Machine

The elliptical machine is a very popular piece of exercise equipment because it combines the motions of walking and running in a virtually nonimpact workout. This workout is designed to increase your cardiovascular endurance while being kind to your body. Because you are doing a repetitive motion, this is a great time to focus on how your body is feeling through the whole range of motion. (Use moving handles, if available, to burn more calories.)

Minutes	RPE	Instruction
1-5	4	Warm-up: Hold on to the stationary handles. Maintain a comfortable pace that allows you to breathe comfortably.
6-8	5	Add moving handles and focus on keeping your abdominal muscles tight.
9-11	5	Hold on to the stationary handles and keep a neutral pelvis.
12-15	5	Add moving handles and allow your heels to lift naturally.
16-18	5	Push the pedals with the balls of your feet.
19-20	4-5	Cool-down: Hold on to the stationary handles as you progressively bring your pace back down to a level that matches your warm-up pace.

Stair Stepper

On this wonderful morning allow your mind to focus on reaching your workout goals. If your goal is cardiovascular endurance and building strength in your legs, then this is the workout for you. As long as you use the stair stepper correctly, this can be an excellent exercise to keep your heart rate up. It is important to keep your body as upright as possible and not to lean forward and put all your weight on the handles. Leaning forward in this way defeats the purpose of this exercise because you don't use your leg strength. Scan your body from your head all the way down to how your feet are positioned on the pedals as you perform this workout.

Minutes	RPE	Instruction
1-5	4	Warm-up: Begin stepping at a slow but steady and rhythmical pace. Strive for a strong vertical posture, allowing your hips and knees to fully extend with each step. Focus on relaxing your shoulders and arms.
6-18	5	Keep your abdominal muscles in tight and allow your legs to do most of the work. Stand upright, focusing on your posture with ears, shoulders, and hips in alignment. Make sure to keep your feet on the pedals.
19-20	4-5	Cool-down: Decrease your intensity. Be aware of keeping your upper postural muscles relaxed.

Stationary Bike

If it's raining this morning or you just prefer riding inside, this is a great way to work out. Because this particular bike workout is an endurance ride, it gives you an opportunity to focus on the mind–body connection.

Minutes	RPE	Instruction
1-5	4	Warm-up: Set your torso in proper alignment by setting your shoulders away from your ears and engaging your abdominal muscles. Begin pedaling at an easy yet steady pace, progressively picking up your speed. Your breathing should be easy at the beginning and get stronger as you pick up your pedal stroke.
6-11	5	Increase intensity a bit. Focus on using a smooth pedal stroke and on working equally with both legs. Continue with this intensity level. Keep your knees over your toes and keep them from swaying from side to side.
12-15	5-6	Push yourself a little harder here. Imagine that you have just begun a slight rolling hill.
16-18	5	You are pulling back just a little to get ready for your cool-down.
19-20	4-5	Cool-down: Bring your intensity down to an easy ride. Not too much resistance here. Imagine you are on flat terrain with little wind resistance.

Rowing

Rowing is a great overall body workout to increase cardiovascular endurance and help build strength in the upper and lower body. Excellent posture and technique are very important when you are rowing. Visualize yourself through each stroke from start to finish. Where are your shoulders? Are your abdominal muscles supporting your low back? How are your feet placed on the foot pedals? Breathe in deeply, clear your mind of any worries, and focus on your breath pattern. Try to keep it as strong and even as possible.

Minutes	RPE	Instruction
1-5	4	Warm-up: 8 to 10 strokes per minute (SPM).
6-18	5	Gradually increase the number of strokes per minute. Keep your abdominal muscles in tight and concentrate on pulling your hands to your shoulders. Get into a rhythm and focus on even and continuous strokes.
19-20	4-5	Cool-down: 8 to 10 SPM.

20-Minute Light Workouts

Jumping Rope

In this light-intensity workout you will intersperse periods of jumping rope (for about 30 to 60 seconds) with various types of aerobic exercises. The goals of this exercise are to build cardiovascular endurance and strengthen the legs and calves. Make sure you have a jump rope that fits your height (see chapter 5 for instructions on choosing a rope). View yourself keeping an erect posture with your chest open and abdominal muscles tight.

Minutes	RPE	Instruction
1-4	4	Warm-up: March in place twirling your rope in circles with one hand.
5-8	5	Place the rope on the ground and pretend you are twirling it with both hands. Alternate jumping lightly with your right foot and then your left foot. March in between if needed.
9	6	Jump rope with alternating feet for 30 to 60 seconds.
10-13	5	Sidestep by jumping from the left foot to the right foot, tapping the left foot to the right after skipping over the rope. Repeat with the right foot.
14	6	Jump rope with alternating feet for 30 to 60 seconds.
15-17	5	Place the rope on the ground and pretend you are twirling it with both hands. Alternate jumping lightly from your right to left foot. March in between if needed.
18	6	Jump rope with both feet for 30 to 60 seconds.
19-20	4-5	Cool-down: Put the rope on the floor and march in place.

Leisure Swimming

Swimming is a wonderful exercise that can be performed in the mornings inside or outside. In this workout, we focus on the front crawl and the backstroke, but if you would like to modify this workout with different strokes that are more suitable for you, go right ahead.

Minutes	RPE	Instruction
1-5	4	Warm-up: Choose your favorite stroke and swim across the pool and back.
6-11	5	Front crawl: Focus your attention on a nice, controlled breathing style.
12-15	5	Backstroke: Keep your navel pulled in toward your spine and relax your neck.
16-18	5	Front crawl: Keep your hands cupped.
19-20	4-5	Cool-down: Swim on your back and kick your legs in a frog-kick motion.

Shallow-Water Walking

If you can find an outdoor pool by your house, this is a great way to start your day. Imagine the warmth of the sun's rays and the cool breeze on your face as you perform this invigorating workout. Using the resistance of the water helps build strength and endurance.

Minutes	RPE	Instruction
1-5	4	Warm-up: Walk across the pool and back swinging your arms at your sides.
6-8	5	Walk across the pool and back reaching your arms alternately up to the ceiling or sky.
9-11	5	Perform the rocking horse in place: Bring your right knee to a 90-degree angle in front of your body and curl your left leg toward your gluteals. Switch sides after 30 seconds.
12-15	5	Do one minute of frog kicks in place, alternating with one minute of cross-country skiing. Frog kick: Jump up with your feet together and knees apart. Push your arms down in front of your body. Cross-country ski: Move across the pool, alternating arms and legs.
16-18	5	Jog lightly back and forth across the pool.
19-20	4-5	Cool-down: Walk across the pool and back moving your arms in a circular motion.

30-Minute Light Workouts

Leisure Walking—Flat Terrain

This walking workout doesn't involve many hills and should be on a flat, curvy path. The goal of this workout is to build cardiovascular endurance. Check the temperature outside first and dress appropriately. You'll want to protect yourself from the sun's rays and bring your water bottle with you.

Minutes	RPE	Instruction
1-5	4	Warm-up: Start at an easy pace; your arms should sway gently forward and back throughout the workout.
6-16	5	Start to increase your pace. Keep full awareness of your posture—your ears, shoulders, and hips should be in alignment and your abdominal muscles should be engaged.
17-21	5	Begin to walk on a diagonal in a zigzag pattern to use different muscles in your feet. Keep your arms close to your body and your elbows bent; do not swing your arms from side to side in front of your body.
22-25	5	Return to walking in a straight line. Pump your arms and continue this pace until the cool-down.
26-30	4-5	Cool-down: Gradually slow down your pace and allow your arms to sway back and forth.

Fitness Walking—Rolling Hills

Hill training is a great workout to increase strength in your legs and calves. You don't have to be a runner to do hill training and gain results. Find a path in your neighborhood that has a couple of hills not more than a 4 percent grade. Focus on the goal of reaching the top of the hill while maintaining a steady heart rate.

Minutes	RPE	Instruction
1-5	4	Warm-up: Start out at an easy pace; your arms should sway forward and back throughout the workout.
6-11	5	Start increasing your intensity on this flat stretch.
12-16	7	Pump your arms and push your legs up the hill. Try to lean from your ankles and not from your hips, and keep your chest open.
17-21	5	Nice and easy down the hill, it's recovery time.
22-25	7	Go back up the same hill—maintain your upright posture and smile!
26-30	4-5	Cool-down: Head back down the hill and let your heart rate slow down.

Road Biking—Flat Terrain

This workout is a great way to wake up, get your workout in, and clear your mind. With this ride your goal is to focus on the pathway of your breath: in through your nose, into your lungs, and then back out through your nose if you can. Focus on the brain–body–breath connection while remaining aware of your surroundings.

Minutes	RPE	Instruction
1-5	4	Warm-up: Scan your body and be aware of your posture. Settle yourself onto your bike and get into a comfortable position. Begin pedaling at a an easy pace with little resistance. Take this time to focus on a smooth pedal stroke, allowing the muscles in your legs to warm up and prepare for the rest of the workout.
6-25	5	Focus on the environment around you. Take in the landscape and breathe deeply while maintaining awareness of the road and traffic surrounding you.
26-30	4-5	Cool-down: Hopefully you were able to breathe in and out of your nose for the whole ride. If not, try to do it now as your heart rate decreases.

Treadmill

This workout is formatted as a cardio circuit and can be performed either walking or running. Your goal is to improve your level of output and power from the first time to the second. Be sure to maintain correct posture throughout the workout.

Minutes	RPE	Instruction
1-4	4	Warm-up: Walk until your core temperature has risen to a working level.
5-7	6	Start pushing yourself a bit harder.
8-9	5	Pull back just a little bit, decreasing your intensity
10-11	6	Increase intensity again. Your breathing will be a bit more apparent here.
12-13	5	Pull it back to catch your breath.
14-15	7	Increase your intensity. This is the peak of your workout!
16-18	5	Recover before the second time through by taking it down.
19-21	6	Here you begin the circuit again!
22-23	5	Decrease your intensity a bit again.
24-25	6	Bring it up a few notches again.
26-27	5	Pull back to catch your breath.
28-30	4	Cool-down: Focus on recovery and even breathing.

30-Minute Light Workouts

Elliptical Machine

Working your heart muscle should be your number one priority every morning. The elliptical machine is a wonderful way to increase your heart rate and get your blood flowing without compromising your joints. Use handles in this workout if they are accessible.

Minutes	RPE	Instruction
1-5	4	Warm-up: Hold on to the stationary handles. Begin by pedaling at an easy and smooth pace, keeping the entire foot on the pedal. Avoid pedaling on only the balls of your feet, as you want to allow all the foot muscles to work through the range of motion.
6-15	5	Add moving handles and allow your feet and legs to move naturally. Push the pedals in a forward motion. Focus on keeping a neutral spine and tight abdominal muscles.
16-25	5	Push the pedals backward. Continue to focus on keeping a neutral spine and tight abdominal muscles.
26-30	4-5	Cool-down: Hold on to the stationary handles and progressively slow down your pedaling to a pace that is close to the warm-up pace. Your breathing should begin to slow down at the end of the session.

Stationary Bike

Sometimes listening to music can help motivate you to increase the intensity of your workouts. Music will help you clear your mind and provide a tempo to which you can synchronize your pedal stroke. This will help keep you from pedaling too slowly. Here is an endurance biking workout that will be good to try with music because you want to maintain the same revolutions per minute throughout the entire ride.

Minutes	RPE	Instruction
1-5	4	Warm-up: Align your torso by sitting upright with chest open and shoulders down, abdominals engaged. Begin to pedal at an easy, light pace while being careful to avoid bouncing in the saddle. Feel the pedals underneath your feet, and make sure your feet are parallel to the floor.
6-25	5	Start to increase your intensity and find a pace that's suitable for you for the entire ride. Choose music with a beat that matches your pace. Keep your back straight and abdominal muscles tight. Relax your shoulders away from your ears and keep your neck long. Focus on positive thoughts.
26-30	4-5	Cool-down: Bring your focus back to your breath.

Stair Stepper

Waking up in the morning and exercising on the stair stepper is a great way to increase or maintain your cardiovascular fitness level. Your body is rested and energy restored, so you can take on this challenging activity! With the stair-stepper workout you'll feel as though you've really worked hard and might even get a good sweat in to help clear your body of toxins. Remember to hydrate before, during, and after your workout. In this workout you focus on cardiovascular endurance and balance.

Minutes	RPE	Instruction
1-5	4	Warm-up: Begin stepping at an easy, yet steady, pace. Set up your alignment by achieving a vertically tall posture—avoid bending forward at the waist. Try not to bottom out (pedals hitting the floor) as you adjust your stepping technique. Keep your chest open and your arms slightly bent.
6-15	5	Increase your intensity with even pedal strokes and try moving your arms forward and back. Keep your abdominal muscles in tight to help you maintain your balance.
16-21	5	Place your hands on the handles. Try not to lean into the machine; your hands are on the handles just for balance. Scan your body from head to toe and align your posture where needed.
22-25	5	Try to take your hands off the handles and pump your arms and focus on your balance.
26-30	4-5	Cool-down: Start decreasing your intensity and continue to do so throughout this interval. Relax your shoulders away from your ears and focus on your breathing pattern as it returns to normal. Feel your muscles respond to the decreased intensity.

30-Minute Light Workouts

Rowing

Whether you are practicing to row a boat or just want a great cardiovascular workout that will strengthen your upper body, this workout is for you. You will be burning about 250 to 350 calories during this workout, depending on your weight. This workout burns more calories than even a bike workout because you are using your upper body and lower body at the same time.

Minutes	RPE	Instruction
1-5	4	Warm-up: 8 to 10 strokes per minute (SPM).
6-21	5	Gradually increase the number of strokes per minute. Keep this pace and focus on pulling your arms and using your back muscles. Press back through your feet and lengthen your legs to full extension. Contract your upper thighs to support your knee joints.
22-25	5	Fill your lungs with air and try to expand your rib cage toward your sides and back.
26-30	4-5	Cool-down: 8 to 10 SPM. Breathe slowly!

Leisure Swimming

Swimming is a great way to burn calories and treat your heart right. The heart is such an important muscle, and moving your arms and legs at the same time will increase your heart rate even more than using just your legs, as in some of the other workouts. Remember that your heart rate is lower in water than it is on land, so make sure you account for this when determining your RPE.

Minutes	RPE	Instruction
1-5	4	Warm-up: Choose your favorite stroke and swim across the pool and back.
6-11	5	Front crawl: Focus on your breathing, and tilt your head to the same side each time to be more efficient.
12-16	5	Backstroke: Lengthen through your arms and legs in each stroke; the opposition should feel as though someone were pulling you from opposite sides.
17-21	5	Sidestroke: Keep your abdominal muscles tight and remember to switch sides after two minutes.
22-25	5	Front crawl: Keep your arm strokes efficient.
26-30	4	Cool-down: Choose your favorite stroke and swim across the pool and back.

Shallow-Water Walking

This workout can be taken inside or outside depending on how you are feeling that day and what the weather is like. Either way, this is a great cardiovascular endurance workout with a variety of moves so that you won't be bored in the water. Focus on using the resistance of the water to help build strength in your arms and legs.

Minutes	RPE	Instruction
1-5	4	Warm-up: Walk across the pool and back swinging your arms at your sides.
6-8	5	Walk across the pool and back reaching your arms alternately up to the ceiling or sky.
9-11	5	Perform the rocking horse in place: Bring your right knee to a 90-degree angle in front of your body and curl your left leg toward your buttock. Switch sides after 30 seconds.
12-15	5	Front kicks: Kick your leg forward while moving across the pool, and push your arms out to your sides through the water. Alternate front kicks with leg lifts: Lift your leg straight back and squeeze your gluteals without extending your low back. Push both arms forward through the water.
16-18	5	Jog lightly back and forth across the pool.
19-21	5	Walk across the pool and back reaching your arms alternately up to the ceiling or sky.
22-24	5	Kick one leg out to the side while punching to the front with the opposite arm. Keep hips square to the front, toes forward, and avoid turning legs out and rotating hips.
25-27	5	Jog lightly back and forth across the pool.
28-30	4-5	Cool-down: Walk across the pool and back moving your arms in a circular motion.

45-Minute Light Workouts

Leisure Walking—Flat Terrain

Walking is one of the best forms of exercise. It is easy to do because you don't need any equipment except a good pair of walking shoes. Scan your neighborhood for different walking paths and streets so that you have a couple of routes to avoid boredom. Being outside with nature can help you feel calm and peaceful and really focus on your exercise goals. This is a flat terrain workout to help increase your cardiovascular endurance. You will need to find walking routes with minimal hills.

Minutes	RPE	Instruction
1-5	4	Warm-up: Start at an easy pace. Your arms should sway gently forward and back throughout the workout.
6-14	5	Always remember your posture: Ears, shoulders, and hips should be in alignment.
15-18	5	Alternate walking on the balls of your feet with walking on your heels in 30- to 45-second intervals. Bend your arms at the elbows and keep them close to your body.
19-25	5	Resume normal walking. Stay light on your feet.
26-31	5	Begin to walk on a diagonal in a zigzag pattern; this makes your inner and outer thighs work harder.
32-39	5	Focus on your mental endurance: You're almost there!
40-45	4-5	Cool-down: Breathe slowly!

Fitness Walking—Rolling Hills

You will want to find a hiking path that is not too hilly or that gives you a nice ascent to start but then levels off or declines in grade. Rolling hills are multiple hills that are pretty even in steepness. The goal of this interval workout is to increase cardiovascular endurance and leg strength.

Minutes	RPE	Instruction
1-5	4	Warm-up: Start at an easy pace; your arms should sway gently forward and back throughout workout.
6-14	5	Start increasing your pace as you approach your first hill.
15-18	7	As you start your ascent, keep your abdominal muscles in tight and your chest open. Watch ahead of you so that you are prepared for any obstacles in your way.

19-25	5	Now you get a little recovery time as you hike downhill. Keep your knees bent and stay light on your feet.
26-31	7	Ascending again, use your leg strength to power up the hill.
32-39	5	Bend at the elbow and swing your arms front to back (each in opposition to the corresponding leg). Swinging your arms will help you maintain your pace and keep your balance as you go down the hill.
40-45	4-5	Cool-down: Breathe and take in the fresh air and the sounds of nature around you as your breathing returns to normal.

Road Biking—Flat Terrain

Make sure your bike is checked out and ready to go. Do you have enough air in your tires? It's best to do this the night before because you'll be getting up early to do your workout. Also make sure to bring a water bottle and patch kit in case you get a hole in your tire. This is a nice, leisurely biking workout. The goal is to increase cardiovascular endurance and enjoy yourself and your surrounding area.

Minutes	RPE	Instruction
1-5	4	Warm-up: Begin by setting up your torso alignment—shoulders down and abdominals contracted. Start pedaling at an easy, comfortable pace, finding a good balance between your pedal stroke and gear setting. Be conscious of your breathing and focus on releasing tension from your shoulders. Begin increasing your pedal speed and adjust your gears (resistance) as necessary. Breathing should be easy and comfortable here.
6-40	5	Maintain an even and smooth pedal stroke. Take in the natural beauty of the surrounding area. Breathe deeply and evenly and be conscious of the muscles in your core, maintaining awareness of your abdominal muscles, shoulders, back, and wrists. Avoid gripping the handlebars too tightly.
41-45	4-5	Cool-down: Breathe as you let your body relax and sink into your seat.

45-Minute Light Workouts

Treadmill

It's time to wake up and get energized for the rest of your day. In this workout you will vary your walking intensity to boost your cardiorespiratory responses. You will want to work as hard as you can on the high points and then let your body recover in between. Internal motivation is key! Forty-five-minute workouts can seem long, but you can do it if you just put your mind to it!

Minutes	RPE	Instruction
1-5	4	Warm-up: Take the time to focus on form as you gradually increase your intensity.
6-10	5-6	Pick up your pace a little bit and focus on your form, taking smaller, more frequent steps. Swing your arms by your sides.
11-15	6-7	Pick up or maintain the pace. Focus on rolling through your entire foot from heel to toe.
16-25	7-8	This is the body of your workout. Your breath should be steady and strong. Take frequent steps at a steady pace. Bend your arms at the elbows, and keep them close to your sides.
26-30	6-7	Bring it down a bit, but maintain a steady pace.
31-35	7-8	Pick it up again—you're almost there!
36-40	6-7	Strong and steady again. Keep the pace—this is the end.
41-45	3-4	Cool-down: Light and easy. Your breathing should be easy yet steady.

Elliptical Machine

The elliptical machine is a great place to get ready for your daily activities. Do you have a problem or concern that you need to mull over? If so, try clearing your mind and focusing on some solutions. When you exercise, your body de-stresses and allows your creative juices to flow. (Use handles if available.)

Minutes	RPE	Instruction
1-5	4	Warm-up: Hold on to the stationary handles as you start at an easy pace.
6-39	5	Add moving handles or try to pump your arms at your sides and work on balance. Keep the rhythm going and let your feet and heels lift off naturally. Push through those legs and pump those arms to get the most out of your workout.
40-45	4-5	Cool-down: Hold on to the stationary handles as you slow the pace down.

Rowing

Imagine rowing down the river and listening to the flowing water on a hot summer day. Feel the warm breeze across your face and imagine yourself steering around the big boulders and rocks that poke out of the water. Clear your mind and focus on integrating the movement between your upper body and lower body. The goal of this workout is cardiovascular endurance.

Minutes	RPE	Instruction
1-5	4	Warm-up: 8 to 10 strokes per minute (SPM).
6-39	5	Gradually increase the number of strokes per minute. Pull your arms back and squeeze your shoulder blades together, keeping your navel pulled in toward your spine. Press with your legs and power through the movement.
40-45	4-5	Cool-down: Breathe and relax your upper body as you slow down to 8 to 10 SPM.

Leisure Swimming

Let your body relax and flow through the water. Try to perform nice, smooth, efficient strokes. This is a leisure swim workout, so try to keep it simple. If you are not as proficient in one of these swimming strokes, then skip it and repeat one of the others that you like better. Remember, this is your workout, so modify it if needed. The goal of this workout is to keep your motions as fluid as possible to complete this 45-minute workout.

Minutes	RPE	Instruction
1-5	4	Warm-up: Choose your favorite stroke and swim across the pool and back.
6-16	5	Front crawl: Keep your breath rhythmic.
17-27	5	Breaststroke: Keep your body in alignment and your abdominal muscles tight.
28-39	5	Butterfly stroke: Try to get full range of motion in your arms and shoulders.
40-45	4	Cool-down: Choose your favorite stroke and swim across the pool and back.

45-Minute Light Workouts

Shallow-Water Walking

Inside or outside, this is the workout for you if you like water or just want to have a great resistance workout as you increase your cardiovascular endurance. The resistance of the water makes this walking activity a great total-body workout and adds variety to your routine.

Minutes	RPE	Instruction
1-5	4	Warm-up: Walk across the pool and back swinging your arms at your sides.
6-8	5	Walk across the pool and back reaching your arms alternately up to the ceiling.
9-11	5	Perform the rocking horse in place: Bring your right knee to a 90-degree angle in front of your body and curl your left leg toward your buttock. Switch sides after 30 seconds.
12-15	5	Front kicks: Kick your leg forward while moving across the pool and pushing your arms out to your sides through the water. Alternate front kicks with leg lifts: Lift your leg straight back and squeeze your buttock without extending your low back. Push both arms forward.
16-18	5	Jog lightly back and forth across the pool.
19-21	5	Walk across the pool and back reaching your arms alternately up to the ceiling.
22-24	5	Kick one leg out to the side while punching to the front with the opposite arm. Keep hips square to the front, toes forward, and avoid turning legs out and rotating hips.
25-27	5	Jog lightly back and forth across the pool.
28-30	5	Walk across the pool and back reaching your arms alternately up to the ceiling.
31-33	5	Perform the rocking horse in place: Bring your right knee to a 90-degree angle in front of your body and curl your left leg toward your buttock. Switch sides after 30 seconds.
34-36	5	Front kicks: Kick your leg forward while moving across the pool and pushing your arms out to the sides through the water. Alternate front kicks with leg lifts: Lift your leg straight back and squeeze your buttock without extending your low back. Push both arms forward.
37-39	5	Jog lightly back and forth across the pool.
40-42	5	Walk across the pool and back reaching your arms alternately up to the ceiling.
43-45	4-5	Cool-down: Walk across the pool and back moving your arms in a circular motion.

60-Minute Light Workouts

Leisure Walking—Flat Terrain

This workout will help increase cardiovascular endurance. You need to find walking routes that do not have hills above a 3 percent grade. Focus on mental clarity and breathing as you walk on this lovely morning. Listen to the wind rustle the leaves of the trees and the colorful birds chirping. Open your mind and think of everything in your life that you are thankful for.

Minutes	RPE	Instruction
1-5	4	Warm-up: Start at an easy pace; your arms should sway gently forward and back by your sides.
6-54	5	Keep your posture upright. Stay light on your feet striking from toe to heel. Try to focus on your gait and rolling off your second toe. Remind yourself to pull your navel toward your spine. Focus on your mental endurance. You can do it!
55-60	4-5	Cool-down: Breathe and relax your muscles.

Fitness Walking—Rolling Hills

Enjoy the morning air on this wonderful hike. Find a curvy path that isn't too difficult but has multiple hills. This is an interval workout to increase cardiovascular endurance and leg strength. Release any tension in your body by scanning it from your head to your toes. Determine what body parts are tight and stretch and relax those muscles.

Minutes	RPE	Instruction
1-5	4	Warm-up: Start at an easy pace; your arms should sway gently forward and back throughout the workout.
6-14	5	Start increasing your pace as you approach your first hill.
15-18	7	Ascend your first hill. Focus on keeping your back straight and not leaning forward from your hips.
19-25	5	Now you get a little recovery time as you walk downhill. Keep your knees bent and stay light on your feet.
26-31	7	Ascending again, use your leg strength to power up the hill.
32-54	5	Bend at the elbow and pump your arms front to back to increase your intensity and maintain the rhythm of your pace. When swinging your arms, make sure they don't cross the midline of your body. Stay focused on the terrain and maneuver around any obstacles in your way.
55-60	4-5	Cool-down: Breathe and take in the fresh air and the sounds of nature around you.

60-Minute Light Workouts

Road Biking—Flat Terrain

The goal of this workout is to increase cardiovascular endurance and maintain leg strength. Safety is very important, so try to pick a trail prior to your workout. Make sure your bike is in good working condition and that you have the proper tools if needed. Don't forget to bring at least two water bottles with you for this 60-minute ride.

Minutes	RPE	Instruction
1-5	4	Warm-up: Stay focused of your whole body and where it is in space as you head out at an easy, rhythmic pace. Begin increasing your pedal stoke toward the end of your warm-up, adjusting your gears as necessary.
6-54	5	Take deep breaths and be aware of the muscles in your core. Try to keep neutral through the wrists and keep a light grip on the handlebars.
55-60	4-5	Cool-down: Relax your whole body, letting it melt into your seat.

Treadmill

Keep up the great work. Some people might already be used to this workload, but others need to work up to this type of endurance. Focus not only on your physical endurance, but on your mental attitude as well. You can do it—just stay focused on your goals.

Minutes	RPE	Instruction
1-5	4	Warm-up: Get your blood flowing and your muscles warmed up.
6-26	5	Swing your arms at your sides. Start to increase the pace to a comfortable rate that you can maintain for 20 minutes. Focus on your body alignment.
27-54	6	Now try to increase the pace just slightly for the rest of the workout.
55-60	4	Cool-down: Light and easy. Your breathing should be easy yet steady.

Stationary Bike

This morning workout will focus on increasing your cardiovascular endurance with light interval training. Don't think of this as hill climbing, but rather as slight increases and decreases in grade. You want to increase your heart rate, and therefore your breathing, just until you would have a hard time finishing a sentence if you were talking. When you're done, relax in your saddle for a minute or two and pedal at a light pace. This additional time will allow you to flush out any lactic acid buildup you may have accumulated during the tougher parts of the workout.

Minutes	RPE	Instruction
1-5	4	Warm-up: Ease into the ride with nice, smooth pedal strokes.
6-14	5	Keep your posture upright: Your ears, shoulders, and hips should be in alignment and your abdominal muscles should be tight.
15-18	6	The grade begins to increase here. Relax your shoulders away from your ears.
19-25	5	The grade decreases. Where is your chin pointing? Keep your head aligned with your spine.
26-31	6	The grade increases again. Keep your elbows soft.
32-54	5	The grade decreases. Great job—maintain this pace. Make sure your knees stay in alignment and point straight ahead and not away from the bike.
55-60	4-5	Cool-down: Relax your body as your heart rate decreases.

60-Minute Light Workouts

Shallow-Water Walking

An early morning water workout is an invigorating way to start your day. It leaves you feeling refreshed, clean, and renewed. In this workout try to focus on maintaining a steady heart rate as you transition from move to move. Fully engage yourself in the moment and pay attention to how each body part moves through the water. Assess the position of your hands. Are they slightly cupped to pull through the water with more resistance? Assess your posture. Are you keeping your abdominal muscles in tight and your chest open?

Minutes	RPE	Instruction
1-5	4	Warm-up: Walk across the pool and back swinging your arms at your sides.
6-9	5	Walk across the pool and back reaching your arms alternately up to the ceiling or sky.
10-13	5	Cross-country ski: Move across the pool, alternating your arms and legs.
14-17	5	Front kicks: Kick your leg forward while moving across the pool and pushing your arms out to your sides through the water. Alternate front kicks with leg lifts: Lift your leg straight back and squeeze your buttock without extending your low back. Push both arms forward through the water.
18-21	5	Jog lightly back and forth across the pool.
22-25	5	Walk across the pool and back reaching your arms alternately up to the ceiling or sky.
26-29	5	Kick one leg out to the side while punching to the front with the opposite arm. Keep hips square to the front, toes forward, and avoid turning legs out and rotating hips.
30-33	5	Jog lightly back and forth across the pool.
34-37	5	Walk across the pool and back reaching your arms alternately up to the ceiling or sky.
38-41	5	Cross-country ski: Move across the pool, alternating your arms and legs.
42-45	5	Front kicks: Kick your leg forward while moving across the pool and pushing your arms out to your sides through the water. Alternate front kicks with leg lifts: Lift your leg straight back and squeeze your buttock without extending your low back. Push both arms forward through the water.
46-49	5	Jog lightly back and forth across the pool.
50-54	5	Walk across the pool and back reaching your arms alternately up to the ceiling or sky.
55-60	4-5	Cool-down: Walk across the pool and back moving your arms in a circular motion.

8

Moderate Workouts

A re you ready to increase your challenge this morning? Do you want to burn more calories, get a little bit more out of your workout, and enhance your aerobic capacity even further? Then choose a workout from this chapter that intrigues you and perhaps allows you to try something a little different. Give your body the opportunity to experience the different routines offered here. Take the time to mentally prepare and focus, incorporating the brain–body–breath connection before, during, and after your session (refer back to the visualization techniques presented at the beginning of chapter 7). This chapter includes moderate workouts for a variety of modalities; they can be performed either indoors or out. Warm-up and cool-down exercises are incorporated into each workout—for recovery workout ideas, please refer to chapter 10. By following the tips offered, you will be able to gain a better understanding of form and alignment as well as the intention of the workout itself.

Other moderate workouts include group exercise modalities such as high- and low-impact aerobics, low-impact power aerobics, step aerobics, circuit training, and aqua aerobics led by certified group fitness instructors at local health clubs or recreational facilities. Chapter 6 reviews some of these options. Your local facility can provide more information, including descriptions of classes and the times they offer them.

20-Minute Moderate Workouts

Fitness Walking—Rolling Hills

This morning workout takes you to the hills! Choose an outdoor area or trail that has various grades in terrain including mild inclines and declines. Parks are usually great for this; however, if there is not a park nearby, choose a route safe from traffic (a residential area with sidewalks works great). Because a normal walking pace is about 15 to 20 minutes per mile (or per 1.6 kilometers), you will probably cover just about that in this workout. Therefore, a 1-mile (1.6-kilometer) route—or a half-mile (0.8-kilometer) route that loops back—would be a good choice.

Minutes	RPE	Instruction
1-5	4	Warm-up: Start at an easy pace, beginning on flat ground. Feel your body adjust to the rhythm of your walk.
6-9	5-6	Increase your intensity a bit, increasing the swing in your arms as you pick up the pace. If you are going downhill, lean back a bit and keep your steps constant to maintain your pace.
10-13	7-8	Find an incline to climb, and lean slightly forward from your ankle joints to work with the hill. Keep the natural rhythm of your arms.
14-17	5-6	Head down the hill (turn around if you are still on an incline) to slow your pace and decrease the intensity. If you are on a decline, use the natural grade to help you decrease your effort.
18-20	4	Cool-down: Bring yourself to flat ground and continue walking, slowing your pace each minute until your breathing is almost normal.

Road Biking—Flat Terrain to a Hill

This morning, let's take your bike to the road! Morning is a great time to get your ride in because traffic is lighter and, in the summer months, mornings are usually much cooler. Because this workout will begin on flat terrain, you probably won't have to go far to find it. However, choose a flat area that offers a bit of an incline; surveying the area before you go might be a good idea. A paved trail or park is bound to offer this kind of terrain. The hill in your workout will build intensity, so focus on continuing to take full, deep breaths as you climb. Maintain a positive attitude as your muscles push you to the top.

Minutes	RPE	Instruction
1-5	4	Warm-up: Easy ride, flat terrain, breathing fairly normally, light resistance, pedals fairly easy to turn.
6-9	5-6	Flat terrain: Pick up speed to increase resistance, or change gears to increase the intensity. Your hill should be in view.
10-13	7-8	Pedal slowly to accommodate the climb, but maintain aerobic effort. Your breathing gets a little heavy here. Change gears, if necessary, to help you climb, and shift your weight back a bit to access your hamstrings more. Hinge at your hips for more of a forward lean, depending on the steepness of the hill, but don't round your back. Keep your torso erect.
14-17	6	Downhill to flat: Bring your torso a bit more vertical as the resistance lessens. Change gears to accommodate the downhill ride.
18-20	4	Cool-down: Find flat terrain to help bring your heart rate and breathing back to normal.

20-Minute Moderate Workouts

Treadmill—Walking and Running

This is a great morning workout for novice and veteran runners alike—in fact, this is a feasible workout for the "nonrunner." New runners, this is a great way to build your base endurance and stamina for running, and you can modify it to be either easy or difficult. Veterans, this is a great recovery workout or a safe way to increase mileage. This workout can be applied to any of the indoor cardiovascular equipment, but it is particularly well suited to prepare you for the challenges of taking your workout to the great outdoors. Outdoors, weather and terrain condition that you didn't plan for can affect your workout. This indoor workout can physically and mentally prepare you for any weather or terrain challenges that may come your way by offering intensity challenges that simulate environmental variables encountered in outdoor workouts. During this workout, focus on the intensity changes as you go from walking to running, then back to walking again. Feel how your muscles and joints respond. Notice changes in your breathing. Take full breaths throughout the workout, concentrate, and never lose sight of your goal! This is a great example of an interval conditioning workout.

Minutes	RPE	Instruction
1-4	4-5	Warm-up: Walk with increasing speed and intention.
5-7	6	Run at a smooth pace that you could continue during a long workout. Your breathing should be even.
8-10	5-6	Walk briskly with your arms pumping. Your heart rate should gradually decrease.
11-12	6-7	Run at a pace that is slightly faster than your last run segment but easy to maintain.
13-14	6	Walk briskly. This recovery time is shorter than the last one, so you have less time to catch your breath.
15-16	8-9	Run at your fastest pace so far. Your breathing should still be even.
17-18	6-7	Recovery walk: This is your last walk interval. Keep it brisk, but your breathing should be heading back to normal.
19-20	4-5	Cool-down: Continue walking, slowing down your pace at 19 minutes and bringing it to a normal walk by the 20-minute mark.

Treadmill and Stair Stepper

This morning workout is perfect on those days that you are on a time crunch. You will work on two pieces of equipment over your 20-minute workout. When you're pressed for time, this workout can maximize your results by increasing the cardio load. Choose two pieces of cardio equipment that you enjoy. One will be for the less intense phase of this workout, and the other will be for a real calorie-burning finish. This workout uses a treadmill for our easier piece and a stair stepper (also called a step mill or stair climber) for the finish. Set the treadmill on manual for 10 minutes; the incline setting is your choice. If you want an easier workout, then keep the incline at 0. If you want to work a little harder, increase the incline to 1 or 2 after completing the warm-up. The choice is yours! Use your brain–body–breath connection to help you decide what will work best for your body this morning.

Minutes	RPE	Instruction
1-4	3-6	Warm-up: Use enough resistance to quickly attain your perceived exertion goal of 3 to 6, walking at a comfortable pace but picking up the pace at minutes 3 and 4.
5-7	7-8	Sprint pace and recovery pace: Alternate 15 seconds of running at an RPE of 8 (sprint pace) with 45 seconds of walking at a recovery pace of 7 to 8. Repeat three times, increasing your effort each time.
8-9	6	Regain composure. Recover.
10-11	6	Transition time to stair stepper: Quickly move from the treadmill to the stair stepper. Set on manual for 10 minutes and begin stepping immediately.
12-13	7	Step with continuous effort at a pace just marginally more intense than walking.
14-16	7.5-8.5	Do 15 seconds at a sprint pace followed by 45 seconds at a recovery pace. Repeat three times, increasing the intensity each time. Don't forget to breathe!
17-18	6	Recover.
19-20	4-5	Cool-down: Reduce the intensity level, feeling your breathing slowing down, your legs feeling heavier, and your steps becoming lighter. Continue until your breathing is back to normal.

20-Minute Moderate Workouts

Stationary Recumbent Bike

If you wake up feeling a bit stiff in your back (perhaps you did a hike or a long run yesterday) or just want to exercise with your back in a supported position, then choose this workout this morning. You will keep up with your cardio activity while giving your torso the support and perhaps rest it needs as you still work the muscles of your lower body. Don't let the position fool you; this is still a great cardiovascular workout. If your bike has a cadence meter, you will want to remain at about 75 to 85 RPM.

Minutes	RPE	Instruction
1-5	3-4	Warm-up: Begin pedaling slowly, increasing your pedal stroke to a resistance that is comfortable and allows you to breathe at a normal pace. Your torso should be upright.
6-9	6	Increase your resistance level until you feel your heel drop. Continue at this resistance level, feeling your leg muscles respond. Your breathing should be a bit heavy. Maintain a constant pedal stroke throughout this level.
10-13	7-8	Increase your pedal stroke for a minute, and then increase your resistance a bit. You will need to slow your pedal stroke down a bit. Feel your breathing respond; your muscles are working harder here. Keep your torso erect, and don't drop your head.
14-17	5-6	Reduce the resistance a bit and increase the speed of your cadence. You should feel lighter in the legs, and your breathing should become a bit easier.
18-20	4	Cool-down: Continue to pedal, a bit slower this time. After one minute, reduce your resistance further until you are at the level you were at during your warm-up. Continue this as your breathing returns to normal.

Elliptical Machine

If you feel the need for a solid aerobic workout without the impact stress to your joints this morning, then the elliptical machine will fit the bill today. If your machine has moving handles, use them because they will add at least 25 percent caloric expenditure to your workout. This workout is quick, challenging, and effective. It will bring attention to your breathing as your legs have to adjust to the changing resistance. Keep that brain–body–breath connection and you will be successful in no time!

Minutes	RPE	Instruction
1-5	3-4	Warm-up: Begin at a low resistance level, pedaling smoothly and keeping your entire foot on the pedal. If you are using the moving arm handles, use light pressure when pushing and pulling them. At this level you can pedal at a constant speed with minimal effort.
6-9	5-6	Increase your intensity. Some machines have a feature that also allows you to increase the angle of the pedal. Raise this a bit if you want to change the target area of your lower leg muscles. Many machines have graphics that tell you which of the lower-body muscles are targeted as you increase and decrease intensity.
10-13	7-8	Increase your resistance level. You will eventually feel your pedal stroke slow down as you adjust to the change in resistance. Keep your body upright.
14-17	6.5-7	Take it backward! Switch your machine to reverse mode and pedal backward. Decrease your resistance level a bit. Shift your weight back a bit to accommodate the change in your center of gravity.
18-20	4	Cool-down: Reverse your pedal stroke back to forward. Bring yourself back to your warm-up resistance level in 15-second increments until your breathing is back to normal.

20-Minute Moderate Workouts

Stair Stepper

Are you in the mood for a hike this morning, but the weather is not cooperating? The stair stepper is the perfect machine to simulate climbing and is a great way to increase the strength in your legs as you build your aerobic endurance. This workout will give you all the challenge of hiking inclines. Envision yourself climbing the foothills of the Rocky Mountains. The steps before you are rocks creating a natural stairway to the top. You are heading straight up, driving your body at a steady pace and building your intensity as you climb. Take a deep breath and focus on your breathing—step by step by step . . .

Minutes	RPE	Instruction
1-5	3-4	Warm-up: Begin by climbing at an intensity that lets you step fairly easily and rhythmically. Your breathing should be fairly normal. Step softly, transferring your weight from one leg to the other and bringing your knee toward your chest, rather than bringing your chest toward your knee.
6-9	5-6	Increase your intensity by increasing your resistance. Be sure to stand tall and not lean on the handles. Make every step count. Go through your full range of motion. Avoid stepping too quickly, which shortens your range of motion.
10-13	7-8	Increase your resistance and feel your leg muscles work as you envision yourself climbing higher and higher. Your breathing should become apparent. You know you are working!
14-17	6	Decrease your intensity level, allowing your legs to feel lighter with each step as your breathing effort slows down a bit.
18-20	4	Cool-down: Continue to climb, but reduce your resistance level until it is similar to your walking level. Your breathing should return to normal. Success!

Rowing

If you are looking for a workout that will work every muscle in your body and leave you feeling exhilarated, then a rowing workout is for you. It is a nonimpact activity that not only uses the muscles in your lower body but also coordinates the use of your upper body with every stroke. You monitor your movements in strokes per minute (SPM); many rowing machine have monitors you can refer to to keep you on track. This morning you will visualize that you are gliding in a sculling boat that takes you across a beautiful lake and back. Although challenging, it is a peaceful, graceful way to meet your aerobic needs today. Refer to chapter 5 for more on rowing technique. If your machine has a pace display, check it often for feedback on how hard you are rowing.

Minutes	RPE	Instruction
1-5	3-4	Warm-up: Row for five minutes very easily, getting a feel for the technique. Aim for a stroke rate of between 24 and 28 SPM.
6-9	5	Continue to row, using your whole body, with more effort, but at a continuous pace.
10-13	6-7	Begin the power 10 sequence: Row with greater intensity (maintaining good form and technique), accelerating the handle toward your body more quickly for 10 strokes at 24 to 28 SPM. Back off and row easily for the next 10 strokes. Alternate these power 10s for the remainder of this time interval.
14-17	6	Row continuously for the next three minutes, focusing on your rhythm and coordinating your arms and legs.
18-20	4	Cool-down: Continue to row, pulling back to a level that matches your warm-up as your breathing returns to normal.

20-Minute Moderate Workouts

Jumping Rope

Rekindle your youth and try this workout that will bring you back to days gone by. Jumping rope is a challenging yet effective activity that enhances heart rate response and agility. It is convenient and inexpensive and can be done anywhere. Grab your rope and your aerobic shoes, and bring energy and excitement to your morning workout today. You will be amazed at how great a workout you will achieve in small amount of time.

Minutes	RPE	Instruction
1-4	3-5	Warm-up: March in place twirling your rope in circles with one hand.
5-8	6	Jump lightly from your right to left foot without the rope first to get used to the footwork action. For the final minute of this phase, pick up your rope and continue the same footwork technique jumping with the rope.
9	8	Jump rope with both feet for 60 seconds. Keep your feet close to the ground and bend your knees each time you land.
10-13	6	Sidestep by jumping from the left foot to the right foot, tapping the left foot to the right after skipping over the rope. Repeat with the right foot.
14	8	Jump rope with alternating feet for 60 seconds.
15-17	6	Place the rope on the ground and pretend you are twirling it with both hands. Jump lightly from your right to left foot.
18	8	Jump rope with your right foot for 30 seconds and your left foot for 30 seconds.
19-20	3-5	Cool-down: Put the rope on the floor and march in place.

Shallow-Water Running

Here's a refreshing way to start your day. Choose this workout when you want to give your joints a rest but still want to get your heart pumping. Find an area of the pool where you can maintain the level of the water from waist deep to shoulder deep. Ideally, your arms should stay in the water. The deeper the water is, the harder your body will have to work against the resistance of the water. The more you work against the resistance of the water, the more strength gains you will achieve in your limbs as well as creating a workload for your heart. As your intensity increases, rely on your brain–body–breath connection to keep your alignment in check as your body is challenged by the resistance of the water. This is surely a total-body workout. Be sure to wear proper footwear as described in chapter 5.

Minutes	RPE	Instruction
1-5	3-5	Warm-up: Walk across the pool and back while pumping your arms forward and back. Your hands can come out of the water, but you will gain resistance if they stay in the water. Increase the pace of your walking at three minutes.
6-9	6	Jog lightly back and forth across the pool. Make sure to come down on your heels and not jog on your toes.
10-13	7-8	Cross-county ski in place: Your legs start together and then split apart—one in front and one behind your body. If you are comfortable with the movement, begin to move back and forth across the pool. Your arms should move in opposition.
14-17	6	Front kicks: Kick your leg forward while moving across the pool. Leap from one leg to the other, raising your leg as high as comfortable while still maintaining your alignment. Alternate punches with leg kicks.
18-20	3-4	Cool-down: Walk across the pool and back swaying your arms in front of you under the surface of the water.

20-Minute Moderate Workouts

Deep-Water Running

If you have access to a deep-water pool, then this workout is worth a try. You will need a floatation belt that can be purchased at sporting goods or swimming specialty stores or on the Internet. In this workout you are suspended in deep water where you will apply the same running movements that you do on land. The difference? Your feet never touch the pool bottom! You will leave feeling refreshed, invigorated, and strong.

Minutes	RPE	Instruction
1-5	3-5	Warm-up: Begin with a progressive yet rhythmic cross-country ski movement with your legs bent and your arms moving in opposition to your legs. Begin with a smaller range of motion and gently increase it. Keep your torso upright.
6-8	6-7	Progress from the cross-country ski movement to knee tucks, pulling your knees into your chest and pressing them straight back down through the water. Alternate these knee tucks with the cross-country ski movement to balance your intensity. Keep your abdominal muscles engaged.
9-10	7-8	Straighten your legs and continue with the cross-country ski pattern, but now with straight legs. Increase the range of motion of your hips as well as your arms. Alternate the position of your hands with palms forward and then palms back as you scoop the water front and back. Alternate the cross-country ski motions with half jumping jacks: moving only your legs in and out with your arms extended out to your sides.
11-13	8	Jog with high knees, sweeping your arms front to back in a circular pattern at chest height with palms down. Focus on keeping your torso erect.
14-16	7	Jog in a straddle position with your knees out to your sides, your hips turned out, and your legs close together. Your arms should be out to the side for balance.
17-18	7-8.5	From a straddle position, increase the width of your legs and alternately raise and lower your knees toward your outstretched arms in a pumping action. You will feel your body create a teeter-totter effect. Keep your torso stable. Emphasize the pushing down action of your legs.
19-20	3-5	Cool-down: Bring your legs back to a normal jogging position and jog gradually, bringing down the intensity and feeling your heart rate return to normal.

Fitness Walking—Rolling Hills

This morning workout takes you to the hills! Choose an outdoor area or trail that includes mild inclines and declines. Parks are usually great for this; however, if there is not a park nearby, choose a route safe from traffic (a residential area with sidewalks works great). Because a normal walking pace is about 15 minutes per mile (or 1.6 kilometers), you will cover about two miles during this workout. You can plan to walk a 1-mile (1.6-kilometer) route twice or walk about 15 minutes out and then turn around and take the same route back.

Minutes	RPE	Instruction
1-5	3-5	Warm-up: Begin walking on flat terrain at a mild yet progressive pace. Perform intervals of walking on your heels and then on your toes. Go back to normal walking, paying attention to your arm position and finding a natural rhythm. Once you are comfortable with your natural rhythm, pick up your pace just a little bit.
6-11	6	Continue to pick up your pace, adjusting your body lean based on the terrain in front of you. When you are approaching a hill, prepare in your mind how you will adapt to that change in terrain.
12-16	7-8	As you begin ascending a mild hill, lean forward from your ankles as you increase your pace. Take smaller steps if necessary, but maintain your speed. Allow your arms to swing naturally with the increased pace, being careful not to let them cross the midline of your body.
17-21	7	Walking down the decline, lean back a bit but stay vertical. Keep the pace; don't allow the grade to push you faster than is comfortable. Don't slap your feet down; focus on the rolling action through your entire foot.
22-25	8	Climb another hill, this time focusing on keeping your chest lifted as you climb. Look straight ahead, not down. Pay attention to your breathing and stay focused. As you begin the descent, slow your pace a bit and feel your breathing adjust.
26-30	5-6	Cool-down: Bring your pace back to the intensity of your warm-up. Feel your breathing come back to normal and the swinging action of your arms slow down.

30-Minute Moderate Workouts

Walking and Running—Easy Hill Repeats

Working on hills is an excellent way to work that derriere. Hills make it easy to keep the heart rate elevated, not to mention the added benefit of improving muscular endurance. Hill repeats are often thought of as super-intense, veterans-only, run-or-ride-til-you-drop kind of workouts. This is not necessarily so. The hill repeat in this workout has been modified so that everyone can get the benefit of the terrain and feel successful. After this workout you'll see how walking on challenging terrain with intention can be just as effective as jogging on a flat road. Choose a hill that is steep enough that brisk walking will keep your heart rate humming. It is also important that the hill be relatively short. A hill that you can see the top of from your starting point at the bottom is preferable. This will allow you to make a few complete repeats before the end of your 30 minutes.

Minutes	RPE	Instruction
1-5	3-6	Warm-up: Walk up your hill, beginning at a normal pace and feeling the intensity increase as you progress through the incline, arms pumping briskly at your sides. When you reach the top, turn around and jog, nice and easy, back to the bottom. Keep track of how many times you went up and back in 5 minutes.
6-10	7	Do the same as before, only now try to increase the number of times you head up and back over the same period of time. Did you add a length—maybe even a lap? If you are up to the challenge, you can also improve your distance traveled by increasing the speed of your downhill jog.
11-15	8	Instead of counting laps, now count how many steps it takes you to reach the top. Continue jogging at an easy pace back to the bottom. Every time you head up, try to decrease the number of steps it takes you to get there, thereby increasing your stride.
16-20	7	Walk at an easier pace on flat terrain, but make sure it still provides a noticeable challenge.
21-25	8-8.5	For the next five minutes you will combine the first two tasks: counting lengths and laps and counting steps. Try to travel the most distance you've covered thus far with the fewest amount of steps thus far (the quickest pace manageable with the greatest strides possible).
26-30	3-5	Cool-down: Progressively jog or walk slower on flat ground for three minutes, slowing your pace down to a normal walk and feeling your breathing return to normal. Continue to walk for two more minutes at an intensity that allows you to breathe normally and evenly.

Road Biking—Flat Terrain to a Hill

Because this workout will begin on flat terrain, you probably won't have to go far to find it. However, because you will want a flat area that offers an incline, surveying the area before you go might be a good idea. A paved trail or park may offer this kind of terrain. The hill in your workout will build intensity, so focus on maintaining full, deep breaths as you climb. Maintain a positive attitude as your muscles push you to the top. This workout is an expansion of our 20-minute workout and is designed to take you a little further, thus enhancing your endurance and leg strength. You will push yourself a little harder and burn more calories in the process.

Minutes	RPE	Instruction
1-5	5	Warm-up: Easy ride, flat terrain, breathing fairly normally, light resistance, pedals fairly easy to turn. Feel your energy at a high at this point.
6-12	6	You are on flat terrain; pick up speed to increase resistance, or change gears to create a bit more intensity. As your hill comes into view, mentally prepare for the challenge.
13-19	7-8.5	Hill climb: Pedal slowly enough to accommodate the climb, but maintain aerobic effort. Your breathing gets a little heavy here. Change gears, if necessary, to help you climb. Shift your weight back a bit to access your hamstrings more. Hinge at your hips for more of a forward lean, depending on the steepness of hill, but don't round your back. Keep your torso erect.
20-24	6-7	Downhill to flat: Bring your torso a bit more vertical as the resistance lessens. Change gears to accommodate the downhill ride.
25-30	3-4	Cool-down: Decrease the intensity by slowing down your pedal stroke on the flat terrain to help bring your heart and breathing rates down. The final minute should find your heart rate returning to normal. Your pedal stroke should be smooth, even, and natural as you return to the pace you had during your warm-up. Your body position should become a bit more relaxed.

30-Minute Moderate Workouts

Treadmill

The following workout is a great way to check your body's ability to recover after a quick start, and it can be done with any piece of indoor cardio equipment. The hardest part of the workout will take place in the beginning as opposed to the end. Therefore, the rest of the workout will be spent coming down from your peak moment. This workout also does an excellent job simulating the start of a race. In a race, you want to surge away from the pack in the beginning and then slowly settle into your pace once you have established your position. This is also a great way to enhance your brain–body–breath connection because you will learn how to push yourself, recover, and maintain reserves to finish strong.

Minutes	RPE	Instruction
1-5	3-6	Warm-up: Use the first five minutes to build yourself to an RPE of 6.
6-7	6.5-7	It's time to mentally prepare for the most challenging phase. Pick up speed and intensity.
8-9	7-8.5	You are pushing the edge of your threshold. You couldn't stay here for too long.
10	8-8.5	Pick up your intensity—this is your peak moment. It's only one minute, so hold strong!
11-12	7-8	The tendency is to come back too quickly—you're still working hard, but nowhere near the edge of your anaerobic zone. Continue to work at an intensity level that is slightly below what you just completed. Concentrate on deep diaphragmatic breathing. You can do this!
13-27	7.5	Now you've reached your pace. You have 15 minutes to remain steady. Stay focused, concentrate. Use your brain–body–breath connection to pull you through. The hardest work is over; now is the time to aim for consistency in your steps as well as your breathing. Strive to keep minute 27 as strong as minute 12.
28-30	3-5	Cool-down: For these three minutes, bring yourself progressively back to a normal pace. Reduce your intensity level each minute, feeling your body and legs respond. Take deep breaths. Bring yourself down to a normal walk as your breathing returns to normal. You did it!

Stationary Recumbent Bike

Feeling the need to get at least a 30-minute cardio workout in, but your body is telling you to pull back a little this morning? Working on the recumbent bike will enable you to keep working toward your cardiovascular goals while giving your torso the support and perhaps rest it needs and still working the muscles of your lower body. If your bike has a cadence meter, you will want to remain at about 75 to 85 RPM.

Minutes	RPE	Instruction
1-5	5	Warm-up: Begin pedaling slowly, increasing your pedal stroke to a comfortable resistance at which you can breathe normally. Grip the handlebars lightly and keep your torso upright. Avoid shrugging your shoulders toward your ears, which can cause neck tension.
6-11	6-7	Pick up your resistance level to the point that you feel your heels begin to drop. Try increasing your pedal speed at each minute. Your breathing should feel a bit heavy. At the 10-minute mark, reduce your pedal speed a bit to get ready for your next resistance change.
12-16	7-8.5	Increase your resistance a bit, focusing on a slower, but steady pedal stroke. Play with the resistance a bit through this interval by increasing your resistance gradually. Keep it steady and strong!
17-21	6-7	Decrease your resistance a bit, and visualize going downhill slightly as you increase your pedal speed. Feel your muscles gain a little more energy with the decrease in resistance. Your breathing should still be a bit heavy.
22-25	5	Focus on pedaling with one leg for one minute, *without* taking your foot off the other pedal. Switch to your other leg for the next minute; then alternate back and forth. For the final minute of this phase, pedal with both legs. Your breathing should be apparent, but not normal yet.
26-30	4	Cool-down: Decrease the resistance further, continuing to focus on the quality of your pedal stroke. Reduce your pedal speed each minute until your breathing is at a comfortable level and you are at an intensity level that matches your warm-up.

30-Minute Moderate Workouts

Stair Stepper

The stair stepper is the perfect machine to simulate climbing and is a great way to increase the strength in your legs as you build your aerobic endurance. Imagine this: You are up early, ready to go, and you have just hit the track at the athletic complex of a college stadium. You have just run around the track for your morning warm-up and now you are ready to hit the bleachers to train for your next performance. Focus on your breathing, close your eyes, and envision yourself ready to take on the stairs.

Minutes	RPE	Instruction
1-5	3-5	Warm-up: Begin by climbing fairly easily and rhythmically. Step softly, transferring your weight from one leg to the other and bringing your knee toward your chest, rather than bringing your chest toward your knee.
6-11	5-6	Increase your resistance. You're climbing higher now. Be sure to stand tall and not lean on the handles. Avoid stepping too quickly, which shortens your range of motion. Step solidly, without bouncing.
12-16	7-8	Increase your resistance and feel your leg muscles work as you envision yourself climbing higher and higher. You can see the top, but there is still a ways to go. Your breathing should become apparent.
17-21	8.5	Hang in there—you are still climbing. Increase the resistance one notch and also speed up your climb. Don't be tempted to lean on those handles or bend forward from your waist: Stay tall. Look ahead, breathe deeply, and stay focused.
22-25	5-7	You are there! It's all downhill from here. Decrease your resistance progressively each minute. Feel your legs respond and your breathing rate even out.
26-30	3-4	Cool-down: Reduce your resistance even further, to a level similar to your walking level. Your breathing should return to normal. Success! Congratulations.

Rowing

If you are looking for a workout that will work every muscle in your body and leave you feeling exhilarated, then a rowing workout is for you. It is a nonimpact activity that not only uses the muscles in your lower body but also coordinates the use of your upper body with every stroke. You monitor your movements in strokes per minute (SPM); many rowing machines have monitors you can refer to to keep you on track. Although challenging, it is a peaceful, graceful way to meet your aerobic needs today. Refer to chapter 5 for more on rowing technique. If your machine has a pace display, check it often for feedback on how hard you are rowing.

Minutes	RPE	Instruction
1-5	3-4	Warm-up: Row for five minutes very easily, getting a feel for the technique. Aim for a stroke rate of between 24 and 28 SPM.
6-16	7-8.5	In this 10-minute time frame, alternate intervals of 40 seconds of harder rowing with 20 seconds of easier rowing. Use the latter part of the 20-second interval as a technique check-in before beginning the next 40-second interval. Row with your whole body.
17-21	7	Use this five-minute time frame to row continuously at a steady pace. Aim for 26 to 28 SPM.
22-26	7.5-8	Repeat the interval drill of 40 seconds of harder rowing with 20 seconds of easier rowing. Keep this going for the entire five-minute time frame. Breathe deeply and keep your focus on your form and timing (refer back to chapter 5) during the slower interval.
27-30	4-5	Cool-down: Continue to row, pulling back to a level that matches your warm-up as your breathing returns to normal.

30-Minute Moderate Workouts

Jumping Rope

This morning, grab your rope and your aerobic shoes and head outside. Because jumping rope can be difficult as a result of the intensity and coordination required for an extended period of time, we have included intervals that allow you to put the rope down and continue the jumping motion without the rope. Feel free to use the jump rope through the entire workout if you desire and have built up the stamina to do so.

Minutes	RPE	Instruction
1-4	5	Warm-up: March in place while twirling your rope in circles with one hand. Engage your abdominal muscles and stand tall.
5-8	6	Place the rope on the ground and pretend you are twirling it with both hands. Jump lightly from your right to left foot.
9	8	Jump rope with both feet for 60 seconds. Keep your feet close to the ground and your arms close to your body.
10-13	6	Sidestep by jumping from the left foot to the right foot, tapping the left foot to the right after skipping over the rope. Repeat with the right foot.
14	8	Jump side to side with both feet for 60 seconds using the rope. Every few jumps, try to draw your knees up to your chest to increase the intensity.
15-17	6	Place the rope on the ground and pretend you are twirling it with both hands. Jump lightly alternating your right and left feet. Keep your hands close to your body.
18	8	Jump rope with your right foot for 30 seconds and then your left foot for 30 seconds.
19-20	6	Place the rope on the ground and pretend you are twirling it with both hands Jump lightly alternating your right and left feet.
21	8	Jump with the rope with both feet for 60 seconds.
22-23	6	Repeat the sidestep, alternating your right and left legs in a side-to-side motion.
24	8	Perform a running step—a slight jog while jumping or skipping over the rope. Avoid jumping high or landing hard.
25-26	6	Place the rope on the ground and pretend you are twirling it with both hands. Skip lightly, alternating your right and left feet. Keep your hands close to your body.
27	8	Begin jumping with the rope with your right foot for 30 seconds; then switch and jump with your left foot for 30 seconds.
28-30	5	Cool-down: Jump with both feet, slowing the turn of the rope down. After one minute, bring it down to a skipping technique, with both feet alternating. For the final minute, place the rope on the floor and march in place as your breathing returns to normal.

Shallow-Water Running

Here's a refreshing way to start your day! Choose this workout when you want to give your joints a rest but still want to get your heart pumping. For this workout, you will need to work in a pool where the water height is at least shoulder level when your feet are in contact with the pool bottom. Ideally, your arms should stay in the water. The deeper the water, the harder your body will have to work against the resistance of the water. Be sure to wear proper footwear as described in chapter 5.

Minutes	RPE	Instruction
1-5	3-5	Warm-up: Walk across the pool and back while pumping your arms forward and back. Increase the pace of your walking at three minutes to increase intensity.
6-9	6	Start to jog at a normal pace. After one minute, perform high knee jogs, bending your knees as you bring them toward your chest; you are aiming for a 90-degree angle at the hip joint. Push your arms down into the water from a bent elbow position at your side.
10-13	7	Cross-county ski in place: Your legs start together and then split apart—one in front and one behind your body. Your arms move in opposition. If you are comfortable with the movement, begin to move forward and back.
14-17	7-8	Straddle jog in place: Your hips are turned out, and your knees lift toward the side. Begin with your arms extended to the side, palms forward; then sweep them back and forth in front of your body, in unison, as you continue to straddle jog.
18-21	7-8	Return to a light jog in place. After one minute, begin to add more intensity by traveling back and forth across the pool as you continue to jog.
22-25	7-8	Perform front kicks across the pool and back, leaping from one leg to the other and raising your leg as high in front of you as comfortable while still maintaining your alignment. Remember to bring your knee toward your chest, not your chest toward your knee. Alternate punches with leg kicks.
26-27	7-8	Do jumping jacks in place for one minute, followed by double jumping jacks for one minute. Double jumping jacks: Jump out to a straddle position, and then jump in place with your legs apart and your arms out to the side. Jump both feet back together, and then jump in place with your legs together and your arms crossed in front of your body.
28-30	4-5	Cool-down: Reduce your intensity with an easy jog for the first minute; then bring it down by walking across the pool and back, swaying your arms in front of you under the surface of the water.

30-Minute Moderate Workouts

Deep-Water Running

This workout offers a variety of movement options in addition to running. You will need a floatation belt that can be purchased at sporting goods or swimming specialty stores or on the Internet. This workout increases your body awareness as you gain cardiovascular endurance and increased strength in your limbs. Because the movements are a bit slower than on land, you can truly concentrate on performing definite actions that require full range of motion. You will leave feeling refreshed, invigorated, and strong.

Minutes	RPE	Instruction
1-5	3-5	Warm-up: Cross-country ski in place with bent legs and each arm moving in opposition to the corresponding leg. Begin with a smaller range of motion, and then gently increase it.
6-8	7	Perform high knee jogs, bending your knees and bringing them toward your chest, aiming for a 90-degree angle at the hip joint. Push your arms down into the water from a bent elbow position at your side.
9-10	8	Perform knee tucks, pulling your knees into your chest and pressing them straight back down through the water. Alternate knee tucks with the cross-country ski movement to balance your intensity. Keep your abdominal muscles engaged.
11-13	7-8	Perform half jacks, pressing your legs out to a straddle position and back. Keep your arms extended out to the side at all times. Alternate slower half jacks with quicker half jacks to vary your intensity.
14-16	7	Run in place while pumping your arms forward and back. Bend your arms at the elbows.
17-18	8-8.5	Move into toe touches: Bring one leg in front of you and reach your opposite hand to your opposite toe. Bring your leg toward your hand rather than bringing your torso toward your leg. Keep your torso erect.
19-20	7-8	To bring down the intensity a bit but maintain the rotating torso action, alternately lift your knees to your chest and reach your opposite hand to your opposite ankle. Again, keep your torso erect.
21-24	6-7	Run in place while pumping your arms forward and back. Bend your arms at the elbows.
25-26	8	Jog in a straddle position, with your knees out to the sides and your hips turned out. Keep your legs close together and your arms are out to the side for balance.
27-28	6-7	Run in place while pumping your arms forward and back. Bend your arms at the elbows. For the final minute of this phase, gradually reduce the intensity of your run and reduce the arm action to a more natural swing.
29-30	3-5	Cool-down: Bring your legs back to a normal running position and run easily, gradually bringing down the intensity.

Fitness Walking Workout

Choose terrain that is moderately challenging: a path with rolling hills, a winding road, or a trail with variable terrain. Variable terrain offers built-in intensity changes.

Minutes	RPE	Instruction
1-10	2-3	Warm-up: Begin walking at an easy pace on fairly flat terrain. Take deep breaths and begin to increase the range of motion in your arms.
11-15	4-5	Begin stepping more quickly in order to increase intensity. Create a V-step pattern by stepping "out, out" and "in, in" to use different muscles.
16-20	5-6	If the terrain allows, walk uphill. If you are on flat terrain, perform a series of 8 to 12 forward lunges followed by 60 seconds of walking.
21-30	7-8	Begin intervals of retro walking—that is, walking backward—preferably on a slight incline. Roll through the ball of your foot first rather than your heel. Pick up your pace as you become accustomed to the action. Alternate two minutes of retro walking with two minutes of traditional walking for eight minutes, finishing off with traditional walking for the final minute of this phase. This is a challenge!
31-40	6-7	Walk forward briskly (becoming aware of your breathing pattern) for nine minutes.
41-45	3-4	Cool-down: Slow your pace down, still maintaining your form and alignment. As in the warm-up, breathe deeply as you feel your heart rate come down a bit and you are walking at a bit more than a leisurely pace. Be sure to take the time to enjoy the scenery and stretch your calves, hip flexors, hamstrings, and low back.

45-Minute Moderate Workouts

Treadmill

This workout will combine walking and running. It is a great workout to jump-start your system's ability to burn calories and train to work at higher intensities for longer periods of time. By using the incline feature on the treadmill, you will simulate changes in terrain. This will naturally result in an increase in intensity, forcing your system to work harder while maintaining your pace.

Minutes	RPE/ Incline	Instruction
1-5	3/0	Warm-up: Begin with a light but brisk walk with your arms at your sides and close to your body and your elbows bent. Focus on rolling through your entire foot. Be conscious of your foot placement and the length of your stride.
6-10	5-6/0.5	Pick up your pace. Increase the frequency of your steps, not the length of your stride.
11-15	7-8/0.5	Begin to run. Try to land softly and keep your arms at your sides and your elbows bent.
16-25	5-6/1.5	Back to a brisk walk.
26-29	7.5-8.5/1	Take it to a run again; this will be a little harder effort interval. Your breathing should be steady yet strong. Keep your strides even and avoid pounding your feet.
30-35	5-6/2	Back to a walk again. Increase the intensity of the walk to keep your heart rate elevated as you back off from running. Your pace is still quick, and you should still be working moderately hard.
36-39	7.5-8/1.5	Back to a run. This is your last effort interval—only three minutes to go!
40-45	3-4/0-1	Cool-down: Your pace should be similar to that of your warm-up. Continue until your breathing is slower and easier and you feel your heart rate has come down significantly.

Elliptical Machine

This workout on the elliptical machine will take you through intervals at intensities that will burn a good deal of calories and condition your heart at the same time. The result of the intervals will be enhanced endurance. If your machine has moving handles, use them because they will add at least 25 percent more caloric expenditure to your workout. This workout will bring attention to your breathing as your legs have to adjust to the changing resistance.

Minutes	RPE	Instruction
1-5	3-5	Warm-up: Begin at a low intensity, pedaling smoothly and keeping your entire foot on the pedal. If you are using the moving arm handles, use light pressure when pushing and pulling them.
6-14	6	Increase your intensity. This should feel steady and rhythmic, but you shouldn't feel as though you are climbing excessively. Some machines have a feature that also allows you to increase the angle of the pedal. Raise this a bit if you want to change the target area of your lower leg muscles. Your breathing should be apparent and conscious, but you should not feel breathless.
15-18	8.5	Increase your intensity until your pedaling speed slows down. If you start to want to hang on to the handles, decrease your intensity a bit. Your breathing should be heavy.
19-24	7	Decrease your intensity to a level similar to that of the prior interval. This is your recovery interval. Your breathing should slow down, but you are still working.
25-28	8.5	Increase that intensity again. This time push it a little further than you did before. The pedal stroke will slow down and should be tough, but still smooth. You can do it!
29-32	7	Decrease your intensity again to that of the previous recovery interval. Your breathing is hard, but steady.
33-36	8.5	Increase the intensity again, but not as high as the last increase. Increase resistance to the point that you feel a change. Simultaneously increase the pedal speed and continue there for four minutes.
37-42	7-8	Switch to reverse mode; then increase your intensity a bit. Feel a slight change in your breathing.
43-45	3-5	Cool-down: Switch back to forward mode. Decrease the intensity to a level that is fairly easy to maintain. Your breathing rate should return to normal with recovery.

45-Minute Moderate Workouts

Stair Stepper

This stair-stepper workout will focus on building endurance for this extended period of time. You will progressively increase your endurance, build to a peak, and then work your way back down. Take a deep breath, close your eyes, and envision yourself ready to take on the stairs: Start stepping!

Minutes	RPE	Instruction
1-5	3-5	Warm-up: Begin by climbing fairly easily and rhythmically. Your breathing should be fairly normal. Step softly, transferring your weight from one leg to the other and bringing your knee toward your chest, rather than bringing your chest toward your knee.
6-14	5-6	Increase your intensity. You're beginning your climb. Be sure to stand tall and not lean on the handles. Avoid stepping too quickly, which shortens your range of motion. Step solidly, without bouncing.
15-20	7-8	Increase your resistance and feel your leg muscles work as you continue to climb. You're not at a peak yet, just at a steady climb. Your breathing is becoming apparent. Keep your pace even and avoid pounding the pedals.
21-29	8-8.5	This is your longest interval. You are working on endurance here. Increase the resistance one notch and also speed up your climb. Keep that form going. Stay tall.
30-35	7.5-8	Decrease your resistance a bit, but keep climbing. You are at a steady pace here, still working on your endurance.
36-41	6-7.5	It's all downhill from here. Decrease your resistance progressively each minute. Feel your legs respond and your breathing rate even out. You are almost there!
42-45	3-4	Cool-down: Reduce your resistance even further, to a level similar to your walking level. Your breathing should return to normal.

Rowing

If you are looking for a workout that will work every muscle in your body and leave you feeling exhilarated, then a rowing workout is for you. This morning visualize that you are on a beach with calm, clear waters. It is early morning; the sun is shining. Out on the open water the only sound you hear are the seagulls overhead and your boat skimming through the water. This morning you will take advantage of the quiet and focus on your form, aiming to make the most of each stroke. Refer to chapter 5 for more on rowing technique. If your machine has a pace display, check it often for feedback on how hard you are rowing.

Minutes	RPE	Instruction
1-5	3-4	Warm-up: Row easily for five minutes, getting a feel for the technique. Aim for a stroke rate of between 24 and 28 strokes per minute (SPM).
6-26	7-8.5	Continue to row steadily and evenly. Every five minutes do a power 10—alternating 10 strokes of greater intensity (keeping your SPM between 24 and 28) with 10 rows of lesser intensity. After each power 10, check your technique before beginning the next one.
27-31	7.5	Row at a steady pace. Aim for 26 to 28 SPM.
32-41	7.5-8	Continue to row steadily and evenly. Repeat the power 10 drill every five minutes. Breathe deeply and focus on your form.
42-45	4-5	Cool-down: Continue to row, reducing your intensity to a level that matches that of your warm-up as your breathing returns to normal.

45-Minute Moderate Workouts

Shallow-Water Running

This workout offers a cardiovascular challenge that strengthens your muscles and joints at the same time. It's an invigorating way to start your day. You will need to work in a pool where the water height is at least shoulder level and your feet are in contact with the pool bottom. Ideally, your arms should stay in the water. The deeper the water, the harder your body will have to work against the resistance of the water. Be sure to wear proper footwear as described in chapter 5. Let's get wet!

Minutes	RPE	Instruction
1-8	3-5	Warm-up: Walk across the pool and back pumping your arms forward and back.
9-14	6	Start to jog at a normal pace. After one minute, perform high knee jogs, bending your knees and bringing them toward your chest; you are aiming for a 90-degree angle at the hip joint. Push your arms down into the water from a bent elbow position at your side. As a variation, swing your arms from side to side, keeping your elbows close to your torso.
15-18	7	Cross-county ski in place: Your legs start together and then split apart—one in front and one behind your body. Your arms move in opposition. If you are comfortable with the movement, begin to move forward and back.
19-23	8	Jumping jacks with reverse arms: Jump from a narrow stance to a wide stance. Keep your arms by your side as you jump out to a wide stance. Move your arms out to the side as you jump back to the starting position.
24-26	8	Do jumping jacks in place for one minute, followed by double jumping jacks for one minute. Double jumping jacks: Jump out to a straddle position and jump in place with your legs apart and your arms out to the side. Jump both feet back together and jump in place with your legs together and your arms crossed in front of your body.
27-31	7.5-8	Straddle jog in place: Your hips are turned out and your knees lift toward the side. Extend your arms to the side, palms forward; then sweep them back and forth in front of your body, in unison.
32-34	8	Jog lightly in place. After one minute, add more intensity by jogging back and forth across the pool. Avoid jogging on just your toes.
35-40	7-8	With both feet together, jump forward and back. Bend your arms at the elbows and keep them stationary as you jump forward and back. Alternate with side-to-side jumps, extending your arms out at shoulder height and keeping them stationary.
41-45	4-5	Cool-down: Jog easily for three minutes; then walk across the pool and back swaying your arms in front of you under the surface of the water.

Deep-Water Running

This workout offers a variety of movement options in addition to running. It will increase your body awareness as you gain cardiovascular endurance and increased strength in your limbs working against the resistance of the water. With a belt on, your body will tend to lean forward more. Make sure it is a *full-body* lean, not from the waist. Maintain an erect torso throughout this workout, and breathe.

Minutes	RPE	Instruction
1-5	3-5	Warm-up: Begin with a rhythmic and easy cross-country skiing movement with bent legs and arms moving in opposition. Begin with a smaller range of motion and increase it gently.
6-10	7	Perform high knee jogs, bending your knees and bringing them toward your chest; you are aiming for a 90-degree angle at the hip joint. Push your arms down into the water from a bent elbow position at your side.
11-18	8	Progress from the high knee jogs to running. Run this entire interval focusing on your form. Maintain a forward, yet tall lean, pulling your knees up and allowing your calves to come up under your hips. Bend your arms at the elbows, and push them through the water in opposition to your legs. Your front arm should come almost to the surface of the water.
19-25	8	Run backward. Face your palms forward and scoop your arms forward in opposition to your legs. Your body is still erect and in the slight forward lean position.
26-30	7.5-8	Perform a cross-country ski action with your legs moving in a scissor-like pattern. Swing your arms forward and back in opposition to your legs.
31-36	8-8.5	Perform half jacks, pressing your legs out to a straddle position and back in with your arms extended out to the side. Alternate slower half jacks with quicker half jacks to vary your intensity.
37-40	7	Run in place with a forward and back pumping action of your arms.
41-45	3-5	Cool-down: Bring your legs back to a normal running position and run easily, gradually bringing down the intensity.

60-Minute Moderate Workouts

Fitness Walking—Rolling Hills

Choose an outdoor area or trail with various grades in terrain. Keeping around a 15-minute pace per mile (1.6 kilometers) will allow you to cover close to 4 miles (6.4 kilometers) in this workout. Find a route that is about 2 miles (3.2 kilometers) in length. You can plan to walk the route and then turn around and take the same route back.

Minutes	RPE	Instruction
1-5	3-5	Warm-up: Walk on flat terrain at a mild yet progressive pace. Perform intervals of walking on your heels and then walking on your toes for three minutes. Go back to normal walking. Once you are comfortable with your natural rhythm, pick up your pace just a little bit.
6-11	6	Continue to pick up your pace, adjusting your body lean based on the terrain in front of you.
12-16	7-8	As you approach a mild hill, lean your body forward from your ankles as you increase your pace. Take smaller steps if necessary, but maintain your speed.
17-21	7	Working down the decline, lean back a bit but stay vertical. Keep the pace, but don't allow the grade to push you faster than is comfortable. Don't slap your feet down. Focus on the rolling action through your entire foot.
22-25	8	Work through another hill or turn around and repeat the hill. Keep your chest lifted and look straight ahead, not down. Begin the descent down the hill; slow your pace a bit and feel your breathing adjust.
26-30	7.5	Working down the decline, feel your body recover a bit. Focus on your heel strike and the rolling action of your foot, being careful not to get ahead of your stride The remainder of the workout will be done on flat terrain.
31-36	8	You will be walking in a V-step pattern: stepping forward and out to the side with both feet and then stepping back to the starting position. However, for this V-step, lower your center of gravity by bending at the knees until you are in a squatting position (make sure your hips don't drop below the knees) as you step out to the side with each foot. Return to a standing position when you step back to the starting point.
37-42	7.5-8	Walk backward (retro walking), focusing on rolling from the ball of your foot through to the heel. If you need to take a rest, turn around and walk normally for a minute and then return to the retro walking when rested.
43-48	7-8	Walk forward at an increased pace. Avoid bending forward from your hips.
49-55	7	Slow your pace down to a moderate walk. After the first minute, alternate walking on your heels and your toes.
56-60	4-5	Cool-down: Bring your pace back to the intensity of your warm-up. Feel your breathing come back to normal.

Walking Circuit

Choose terrain that is moderately challenging: a path with rolling hills, a winding road, or a trail with variable terrain. Variable terrain offers built-in intensity changes.

Minutes	RPE	Instruction
1-10	2-3	Warm-up: Begin walking at an easy pace on fairly flat terrain. Take deep breaths and begin to increase the range of motion of your arms.
11-15	4-5	Begin stepping more quickly in order to increase intensity. You will be walking in a V-step pattern: stepping forward and out to the side with both feet and then stepping back to the starting position. However, for this V-step, lower your center of gravity by bending at the knees until you are in a squatting position (make sure your hips don't drop below the knees) as you step out to the side with each foot. Return to a standing position when you step back to the starting point.
16-20	5-6	If the terrain allows, walk an incline. If you are on flat terrain, perform a series of 8 to 12 forward lunges followed by 60 seconds of walking.
21-30	7-8	Begin intervals of retro walking, preferably on a slight incline. Roll from the ball of your foot first rather than from your heel. Pick up your pace as you become accustomed to the action. Alternate two minutes of retro walking with two minutes of traditional walking for eight minutes, finishing off with traditional walking for the final minute of this phase. This is a challenge!
31-40	6-7	Walk forward briskly, becoming aware of your breathing pattern.
41-45	7.5-8	Perform a series of 8 to 12 forward lunges followed by 60 seconds of walking.
46-51	7.5	Repeat the V-step pattern.
52-55	7	Walk normally, keeping a quick pace to maintain your intensity.
56-60	4-5	Cool-down: Slow your pace down. Breathe deeply as you feel your heart rate come down.

60-Minute Moderate Workouts

Road Biking—Flat Terrain to a Hill

Today your focus will be on gaining endurance and building stamina in your legs to train for longer rides. Let's get rolling! Choose a flat area that offers a bit of an incline, such as a paved trail or park. Because the hill in your workout will build intensity, focus on maintaining full, deep breaths as you climb. Keep your attitude positive as your muscles push you to the top.

Minutes	RPE	Instruction
1-5	5	Warm-up: Easy ride, flat terrain, breathing fairly normally, light resistance, pedals fairly easy to turn.
6-14	6	Flat terrain: Pick up speed to increase your intensity, or change gears to create resistance, but keep the speed constant. At 10 minutes, maintaining the same resistance, pedal a bit faster. Stay at this cadence for one minute; then repeat by increasing your pedal speed about 5 to 10 percent each minute for three minutes.
15-19	7.5-8.5	Hill climb: Use a slower pedal stroke and adjust your gears to accommodate the climb but maintain aerobic effort. Your breathing should get a little heavy here. Keep your torso erect.
20-27	7	Downhill to flat: As your resistance lessens, change gears to accommodate the downhill ride. Once on flat ground, continue to pedal at a constant speed, adjusting your gear speed to allow you to keep a steady pedal speed. Your breathing should be steady and aerobic.
28-33	7.5-8.5	Hill climb: Use a lower pedal stroke, adjusting your gears to accommodate the climb but maintain aerobic effort. Your breathing gets a little heavy here. Change gears, if necessary, to help you climb the hill. Keep your torso erect.
34-41	7	Downhill to flat: As resistance lessens, change gears to accommodate the downhill ride. Once on flat ground, continue to pedal at a constant speed, adjusting gear speed to allow you to keep a steady pedal speed. This is your road pace. Pedal consistently without gliding.
42-48	8	You should be on flat terrain for the remainder of the workout. Every two minutes, increase the speed of your legs by 5 to 10 percent. If you encounter mild inclines, adjust your pedal speed accordingly to accommodate the changing terrain, but try to maintain a speed higher than the previous two minutes.
49-52	7.5	Decrease your speed, feeling your legs recover.
53-60	4-5	Cool-down: Decrease your intensity by slowing down your pedal stroke. During the final minute, return to your warm-up pace.

Treadmill

In this workout the incline feature on the treadmill simulates changes in terrain. This will naturally result in an increase in intensity, forcing your system to work harder while you maintain a strong and steady pace. You will be amazed how intervals can make your time fly!

Minutes	RPE/ Incline	Instruction
1-5	3/0	Warm-up: Walk lightly but briskly with your arms at your sides and close to your body, your elbows bent. Roll through your entire foot.
6-10	5-6/0	Pick up your pace. Increase the frequency of your steps, not the length of your stride.
11-15	7-8/0	Begin to run. Land softly and keep your arms at your sides, with your elbows bent. Your breathing should be steady.
16-25	8/1	Continue to run. Maintain the same pace as your last interval. Don't let the incline slow you down.
26-28	8-8.5/2	Continue to run. Your breathing should be steady yet strong. Take even strides and avoid pounding your feet.
29-32	7.5/0	Recovery interval with no incline. This should feel a bit easier, but your breathing should still be apparent.
33-34	8-8.5/1.5	Back to a running on an incline. Maintain a steady pace.
35-36	8.5/2.5	The incline gets steeper. Lean forward to accommodate the change in terrain.
37-41	7.5/0.5	Recovery interval: Continue running at a more comfortable pace. You should still be breathing hard and working.
42-45	8/2.5-3	Another incline. Feel your body naturally lean forward to adjust to the change in terrain. Your pace may slow down a bit; that's OK, just keep it steady.
46-49	7.5/0.5	Recovery interval. You are running at a normal running pace, still working, but recovering from your last effort interval.
50-51	8.5/3	Give it your all! This is a one-minute uphill climb. Keep everything in check and focus on your form.
52-60	4-5/0	Cool-down: Your pace should be similar to that of your warm-up. Continue until your breathing is slower and easier and your heart rate has come down significantly.

60-Minute Moderate Workouts

Stationary Recumbent Bike

Working on the recumbent bike will enable you to keep working toward your cardiovascular goals—working the muscles of your lower body while giving your torso the support and perhaps rest it needs. Don't let the position fool you; this is a great cardiovascular workout. If your bike has a cadence meter, you will want to remain at about 75 to 85 RPM.

Minutes	RPE	Instruction
1-5	5	Warm-up: Begin pedaling slowly, increasing your pedal stroke to a resistance that is comfortable and allows you to breathe at a normal pace.
6-13	6-7	Increase your resistance level until you feel your heels begin to drop. Try increasing your pedal speed at each minute. At the 12-minute mark, reduce your pedal speed a bit to get ready for your next resistance change.
14-20	7-8.5	Increase your resistance gradually in one-minute increments. For the last two minutes, find a resistance level at which you can feel your hamstrings working and still keep a steady pace You should be conscious of your breathing.
21-28	6-7	Decrease your resistance a bit. Feel your muscles gain a little more energy with the decrease. Your breathing should be steady. Alternate short periods of quicker speed bursts.
29-34	6	Focus on pedaling with one leg and then the other for two-minute intervals *without* taking your nonpedaling foot off the pedal. For the final minute of this phase, pedal with both feet. Your breathing should be apparent, but you should not be breathless.
35-41	7-8	Endurance ride: Increase your resistance until you feel your heels drop and your hamstrings kick back in. Focus on maintaining a constant pedal stroke and speed.
42-45	8	Increase your resistance to simulate a slight incline. Increase the resistance only until you feel a slight change; don't push so hard that your stroke becomes uneven. Slow your pedal stroke down a bit and keep it steady, smooth, and strong.
46-49	7.5	Decrease the resistance to simulate flat terrain. Increase your pedal speed and maintain a steady stroke.
50-53	8	Decrease your pedal speed and increase the resistance for a final push. This is your last effort before you cool down. Keep your pedal stroke even and be careful not to rock from side to side with your body.
54-57	6-7	Bring your resistance down to where you can pedal easily without strain. Your breathing should be returning to normal, but you are still working.
58-60	4-5	Cool-down: Decrease your resistance. Reduce your pedal speed each minute until your breathing is at a comfortable level and your intensity level matches that of your warm-up.

Elliptical Machine

This workout will take you through intervals at intensities that will burn a good deal of calories, condition your heart, and enhance your endurance levels. If your machine has moving handles, use them because they will add at least 25 percent more caloric expenditure to your workout. Be careful not to put your weight into the handles.

Minutes	RPE	Instruction
1-5	3-5	Warm-up: Begin at a low intensity, pedaling smoothly and keeping your entire foot on the pedal. If you are using the moving arm handles, use light pressure when pushing and pulling them.
6-14	6	Increase your intensity. This should feel steady and rhythmic, but you shouldn't feel as though you are climbing excessively. Your breathing should be apparent and conscious, but you should not be breathless.
15-18	8.5	Increase your intensity until your pedaling speed slows down. If you find you want to hang on to the handles, decrease your intensity a bit. Your breathing should be heavy.
19-24	7	Decrease your intensity to a level similar to that of the prior interval. This is your recovery interval. Your breathing should slow down, but you are still working.
25-28	8.5	Increase that intensity again. This time push it a little further than you did before. The pedal stroke will slow down and should be tough, but still smooth.
29-34	7	Decrease to a level where you can sustain a rhythmic, aerobic pace similar to that of an endurance workout. Your breathing should be hard, but steady.
35-38	8	Increase the intensity again, but not as high as last time. In this interval you want to work on speed *with* resistance, so increase the resistance to the point that you feel a change. Once you have adjusted to the increase in resistance, you can increase the pedal speed.
39-44	8-8.5	Switch to reverse mode and increase your intensity a bit. You will have to shift your weight back a bit here to adjust for the change in pedal position. However, don't lose your vertical position.
45-48	7.5-8	Switch to forward mode. Keep the resistance at the same level. Your breathing should be apparent and strong.
49-52	8	Increase your resistance. You're breathing harder now. Take deep breaths—you are in the final stretch.
53-56	7-7.5	Decrease your intensity enough to allow your breathing to slow down a bit and recover. Feel your body and breathing become comfortable but steady.
57-60	3-5	Cool-down: Decrease the intensity to a level that is fairly easy to maintain. Continue to decrease your intensity in 30-second to one-minute intervals until you are at your warm-up level. Your breathing should return to normal levels.

60-Minute Moderate Workouts

Shallow-Water Running

This workout offers a cardiovascular challenge that strengthens your muscles and joints at the same time. You will need to work in a pool where the water height is at least shoulder level and your feet are in contact with the pool bottom. Ideally, your arms should stay in the water. The deeper the water, the harder your body will have to work against the resistance of the water. Be sure to wear proper footwear as described in chapter 5.

Minutes	RPE	Instruction
1-8	3-5	Warm-up: Walk across the pool and back pumping your arms forward and back. Increase the pace of your walking at three minutes to increase intensity.
9-14	6	Start to jog at a normal pace. After one minute, perform high knee jogs, bending your knees and bringing them toward your chest; you are aiming for a 90-degree angle at the hip joint. Push your arms down into the water from a bent elbow position at your side. As a variation, swing your arms from side to side, keeping your elbows close to your torso.
15-18	7	Cross-county ski in place: Your legs start together and then split apart—one in front and one behind your body. Your arms move in opposition. If you are comfortable with the movement, begin to travel back and forth across the pool.
19-23	8	Jumping jacks with reverse arms: Jump from a narrow stance to a wide stance, keeping your arms at your sides. Move your arms out to the side as you jump back to the starting position.
24-26	8	Do jumping jacks in place for one minute, followed by double jumping jacks for one minute. Double jumping jacks: Jump out to a straddle position, and then jump in place with your legs apart and your arms out to the side. Jump both feet back together, and then jump in place with your legs together and your arms crossed in front of your body.
27-31	7.5-8	Straddle jog in place: Your hips are turned out and your knees lift toward the side. Extend your arms to the side, palms forward; then sweep them back and forth in front of your body, in unison.
32-34	8	Jog lightly in place. After one minute, add more intensity by jogging back and forth across the pool. Avoid jogging on just your toes.
35-40	7-8	With both feet together, jump forward and back. Bend your arms at the elbows and keep them stationary as you jump forward and back. Alternate with side-to-side jumps in which you hold your arms stationary as you extend them out at shoulder height.
41-45	7.5-8.5	Jog or run in place for two minutes. Then, immerse yourself up to your shoulders. Keeping this lower center of gravity, pick up your pace and run harder and more vigorously for 60 seconds. Follow with 60 seconds of running in the original upright position and then 60 seconds of immersed running.

46-50	8	Run across the pool and back for five minutes pumping your arms.
51-55	7	Jog across the pool and back. After one minute, perform high knee jogs, bending your knees and bringing them toward your chest, aiming for a 90-degree angle at the hip joint. Push your arms down into the water from a bent elbow position at your side.
56-60	4-5	Cool-down: Do an easy jog across the pool. After three minutes, walk across the pool and back swaying your arms in front of you under the surface of the water.

Deep-Water Running

This workout offers a variety of movement options in addition to running. It will increase your body awareness as you gain cardiovascular endurance and increased strength in your limbs working against the resistance of the water. With a belt on, your body will tend to lean forward more. Make sure it is a *full-body* lean, not from the waist. Maintain an erect torso throughout this workout, and breathe.

Minutes	RPE	Instruction
1-5	3-5	Warm-up: Begin with a rhythmic and easy cross-country skiing movement with bent legs and arms moving in opposition to the legs. Begin with a smaller range of motion and increase it gently.
6-10	7	Perform high knee jogs, bending your knees and bringing them toward your chest, aiming for a 90-degree angle at the hip joint. Push your arms down into the water from a bent elbow position at your side.
11-18	8	Progress from the high knee jogs to running. Run this entire interval focusing on your form. Maintain a forward, yet tall lean, pulling your knees up and allowing your calves to come up under your hips. Bend your arms at the elbows and push them through the water in opposition to your legs. Your front arm should come almost to the surface of the water.
19-25	8	Run backward. Face your palms face forward and scoop your arms forward in opposition to your legs. Your body should still be erect and in the slight forward lean position.
26-30	7.5-8	Perform a cross-country ski action with your legs moving in a scissor-like pattern. Swing your arms forward and back in opposition to your legs.
31-36	8-8.5	Perform half jacks, pressing your legs out to a straddle position and back in with your arms extended out to the side. Alternate slower half jacks with quicker half jacks to vary your intensity.
37-40	7.5-8	Run in place with a forward and back pumping action of the arms.

(continued)

60-Minute Moderate Workouts

41-47	8	Run backward. Face your palms forward and scoop your arms forward in opposition to your legs. Your body should still be erect and in the slight forward lean position.
48-51	8	Perform high knee jogs, bending your knees and bringing them toward your chest, aiming for a 90-degree angle at the hip joint. Push your arms down into the water from a bent elbow position at your side.
52-55	7	Run in place with a forward and back pumping action of the arms.
56-60	3-5	Cool-down: Bring your legs back to a normal running position and run easily, gradually bringing down the intensity.

9

Intense Workouts

Are you ready for some workouts that will take your heart rate to the max? Then these workouts are for you. This chapter outlines a variety of intense workouts in a variety of modalities designed to enhance your cardiorespiratory response and burn significant calories. These workouts will train your system to work at higher intensities for longer periods of time, thereby increasing your aerobic capacity. They are geared toward people already engaged in aerobic exercise routines on a regular basis. As with the workouts in other chapters, it is important to mentally prepare and focus on each one, incorporating the brain–body–breath connection before, during, and after your session (refer back to the visualization techniques presented at the beginning of chapter 7). Warm-up and cool-down exercises are again incorporated into each workout—for recovery workout ideas, please refer to chapter 10.

20-Minute Intense Workouts

Running

This workout has two separate phases. Your goal is to improve from the first phase (minutes 5-12) to the second phase (minutes 13-20). Designate a long set of stairs (stadiums are great for this), a track, or any measurable hill or street that makes it easy to keep track of your "laps." A hill or stairs will build leg strength, whereas a track will build cardiovascular endurance. Your start and end point should be the same.

Minutes	RPE	Instruction
1-4	3-5	Warm-up: Begin running, focusing on your form and breathing.
5-10	6-8.5	Start counting your laps now. Increase your pace progressively each minute until you feel a change both in your breathing and muscle activation. You should be breathing hard here.
11-12	7	March in place for 60 seconds. This is your only recovery.
13-18	8.5	Your goal in this interval is to add more laps, even if it's just one or a half. Start counting your laps. Increase your pace again, pushing until you feel your breathing respond heavily but you can still keep your alignment and technique in check. Breathe deeply and set your mind on the task at hand.
19-20	3-6	Cool-down: Bring your pace down to a walk, allowing your breathing to return to normal.

Running—Speed Work

This workout focuses on increases in speed. Speed work should only be done once or twice a week, *at the most.* Because you will take longer to recover from a speed workout than from a regular workout, if you do them too often, you can undermine your progress. You should attempt speed workouts only once you have achieved a good base level of cardiovascular endurance. If running is not your game, this workout can be applied to lap swimming or outdoor cycling. A track is the perfect place to do speed work because you can see your end point and measure your improvement. If a track is not available, any stretch of measurable road will do the trick. You will need a longer recovery from this workout than you will from the previous 20-minute running workout. By using your recovery period wisely, you will enhance your body's ability to take up oxygen, which in turn will greatly improve your endurance. Sometimes adding speed workouts to your routine is all it takes to break out of a workout plateau.

20-Minute Intense Workouts

Minutes	RPE	Instruction
1-4	3-5	Warm-up: Begin jogging lightly, progressing to a gentle run. Establish correct technique and form here.
5-6	8-8.5	Increase frequency of your steps to increase your intensity. Pump your arms faster by your sides. You should be breathing hard here.
7-8	6-7	Return to a lighter jog, decreasing your intensity by decreasing the frequency of your steps. This is your active recovery. Feel your breathing lighten up a bit, although you are still working here. During the last 30 seconds, mentally prepare for the next interval, which you will perform at a much higher intensity.
9-9:30	9	Pick up your pace here and *sprint!* You should be breathless at this point. Notice the distance you travel during this interval because you will want to go a little farther on the next high-effort interval.
9:31-11	6	Bring it down to a walk. This is your active recovery—catch your breath.
12-15	6.5-7.5	Increase your intensity to a light run (your RPE should be about 7.5). Because of the high intensity of the sprint interval you just finished, your perceived exertion might feel greater in this interval than it did when you performed your light jog during the warm-up. As you get to a steady pace, your actual perceived exertion will come down a bit from the beginning of the last interval. Mentally prepare for your next interval.
16-16:30	9	Sprint again. Your goal is to travel farther than you did in your last sprint. You should be breathless again here.
16:31-17:30	6	Return to a walk. Your heart rate should come down a bit. Prepare for the next sprint.
17:31-18	9	Sprint again, trying to travel farther than you did in the last sprint. If you can't, just try to maintain the pace you had in the previous sprints. You should be breathless here.
19-20	6	Cool-down: Walk. Let your heart rate come down completely, and feel your breathing come back to normal. You might want to take a few more minutes here to cool down if you need more time. Your blood pressure will return to normal and you can give your lungs the opportunity to get back into their natural breathing rhythm.

20-Minute Intense Workouts

Race Cycling

In this short, but challenging workout you will take to the open road and work on speed. Find a road that is fairly flat. A slight incline or grade will not hinder the workout; it will just make it a bit more challenging in those sections. You are going to race against yourself this morning, working on speed and trying to cover as much distance as possible.

Minutes	RPE	Instruction
1-5	5	Warm-up: Begin cycling at a speed that is easy to maintain. Focus on a smooth pedal stroke and maintaining an erect torso.
6-8	7-7.5	Begin to increase your pedal stroke. If necessary, increase your resistance or change gears to avoid bouncing in the saddle. At minute 7 increase your pedal stroke again to drive yourself to cover more ground. Keep this pace for the next two minutes.
9-10	9	Sprint for this interval, not until you are completely breathless and out of oxygen but until you find it hard to speak in a full sentence.
11-12	7	Reduce your speed to recover, maintaining a pace that is manageable but still feels like work. Your breathing should be apparent, but you should be able to cycle with ease.
13-14	8-8.5	Increase your speed until you feel your heart rate increase and your muscles respond. Your breathing should become heavier.
15-16	9	Increase your speed to a sprint! Cover as much ground as possible—it's only a minute, so hang in there.
17-18	7	Reduce your speed to recover. Allow your breathing to ease off.
19-20	4-6	Cool-down: Continue to reduce your speed until you are at an intensity that is equal to that of your warm-up. Pedal until your breathing comes back to normal and your legs feel lighter.

Treadmill

This workout is designed to push you to the limit to take you to the next level of fitness. Often the only difference between a moderate and an intense workout is the ability to push your mental endurance. Getting past what at first you thought was too difficult or impossible is what puts you a cut above the rest and improves your physique and your mental game. To truly make this workout effective, you must have a solid base level of aerobic fitness and be willing to push into the realms of discomfort. Because this workout is short, you must increase the intensity to meet your goals. This is done using varying inclines to simulate variety in terrain. As you get stronger, you can increase the grade, or you can set your speed higher. These challenges, as tough as they are, will provide the most fitness gains.

Minutes	RPE/ Incline	Instruction
1-5	3-6/0	Warm-up: Start jogging at a comfortable pace. You are establishing the speed you will maintain during the entire workout, so find one you can commit to.
6-8	7/1.5	Try to maintain the same pace. You are at a normal jog or run, breathing harder but comfortable in your stride. If you feel your heart rate is increasing too rapidly, decrease the grade but maintain your speed. Focus on correct form here.
9-11	7.5/2.0	Increase the incline again here, but focus on maintaining the same pace. As the incline increases, you may feel the need to lean a bit forward. Make sure you lean from your ankles and not from your waist.
12-14	8-8.5/3.5	Increases the incline once more. This is the most difficult increase, and you will feel yourself pushing further toward your peak. Your breathing should be heavy and quite apparent. Don't lose your form or your pace.
15-16	6.5-7/0	Maintain the same pace. You will want to slow down, but stay committed to the pace you have been working at. Maintain good posture and concentrate on landing softly.
17-18	8.5-9/4	This is the peak! Maintain the same pace as before. Let yourself fall naturally into a full-body lean. Oxygen is your fuel—take it in and finish solid!
19-20	4-6/0	Cool-down: Walk briskly at a pace that gradually slows down.

20-Minute Intense Workouts

Treadmill—Steep Hill Simulation

This workout will allow you to burn a significant amount of calories as well as give your legs a heavy workout in a short amount of time. You will be working on a treadmill, simulating a steep climb. Focus on your form as you begin and continue to climb. Because your body lean will be more forward, this workout will specifically work the gluteals, quadriceps, and hamstrings. In addition you will gain improved core strength and stabilization as the abdominals and back muscles will have to work together to keep your torso in proper alignment. Breathe deeply and commit to the workout. Start climbing!

Minutes	RPE/ Incline	Instruction
1-5	3-5/0	Warm-up: Walk at a normal pace preparing both mentally and physically for the workout. At minute 3 pick up your pace, feeling both your body and breathing respond. Roll naturally from the heel of your foot through to the ball of your foot. Bend your elbows and keep them close to your sides.
6-8	6-6.5/0	Pick up the pace even more, feeling your breathing respond and your arm swing increase.
9-10	7-7.5/1	Increase your incline to 1 percent. Try to maintain the same pace as the last interval.
11-13	8/2.5	Increase your incline to 2.5 percent. If you can, try to increase your speed by .5 mph. Maintain a forward lean from your ankles only. Avoid leaning forward from your waist. Keep your torso erect.
14-16	8.5/3-3.5	Prepare your mind and body to climb again. Increase your incline without decreasing your pace. Feel your breathing get heavier, but you should not be breathless. Allow your arms to swing naturally by your sides; do not swing them across the midline of your body. You can do this!
17-18	9/3.5-4	Increase your pace, increase the incline to 4 percent, or both. Deep breaths are required. Try to increase the frequency of your steps rather than the length of your stride. Still maintain your heel, ball, toe technique. This is only one minute; hang in there!
19-20	6	Cool-down: You made it! Drop your incline down gradually as well as your mph. Your legs should feel lighter as your breathing comes back to normal levels.

Treadmill—Race Walking

This workout uses race walking techniques as you take on the challenge of a steep hill climb. Your goal is to race walk to the top of a simulated hill, maintaining a race walk pace throughout. Race walking techniques are reviewed in chapter 4. A quick review of those techniques will reinforce in your body and mind the ideal foot strike and body position necessary to get you through this short, yet effective workout. Taking smaller, quicker, and more frequent steps rather than increasing your stride will work best here to maintain the hip rotation required to keep up your pace. On your mark, get set . . . let's go!

Minutes	RPE/ Incline	Instruction
1-5	5/0-.5	Warm-up: Take a deep breath, focus, and begin your climb. Start at a normal walking speed, but quickly move into your correct race walking technique. At minute 3 increase your incline to .5 percent.
6-9	7-7.5/1	Continue to race walk, progressively increasing your steps as you move into the body of the workout. Your breathing should be getting heavy here. Maintain the rolling action from the heel to the ball of your foot and through to the push-off. Let the hip rotation occur naturally as you continue to place your feet along a straight line. Pump your arms back and forth without letting them cross the midline of your body.
10-13	8-8.5/2	Increase the frequency of your steps, not your stride. Maintain your rhythm and hip rotation at this increase. Avoid slapping the balls of your feet on the ground.
14-16	8.5-9/2.5-3.5	Every 30 seconds increase your incline by .5 percent. Feel your body lean from your ankles. Stay vertical and erect. Take smaller steps if necessary, but maintain your pace. Your breathing should be very apparent at this point. Use those arms swinging from the shoulders to keep you going.
17-20	5-7/.5-3.5	Cool-down: Progressively at 30-second intervals, reduce your incline. At minute 19 you should be at .5 percent or less. Bring your pace down to a normal walk and allow your breathing to come back to normal.

20-Minute Intense Workouts

Rowing

Rowing works every muscle in your body and leaves you feeling exhilarated. The best part is that it is a nonimpact activity that enhances the coordination of your body as a whole. You will work in five-minute intervals and get a complete, intense, and challenging workout that will prepare you for longer rowing workouts to come. This short, yet effective workout will test your ability to maintain consistent and efficient strokes. Aim for 26 to 28 strokes per minute (SPM). Refer to chapter 5 for rowing technique tips.

Minutes	RPE	Instruction
1-5	5	Warm-up: Row very easily, getting a feel for the technique. Aim for a stroke rate of between 24 and 28 SPM.
6-10	7	Continue to row, using your entire body at a moderate yet challenging pace of 26 to 28 SPM. During the last minute mentally prepare for your first interval of power 10s.
11-15	8.5	Power 10 intervals: Every minute perform 10 strokes at a greater intensity followed by 10 strokes at a lesser intensity. To do this, you will need to use your legs, back, and arms to pull the handle toward your body more quickly. Each power 10 should be with greater intensity than the one before. Row at a steady pace between power 10 intervals.
16-18	7.5-8	Row at a moderate yet challenging pace. During the last minute, row with greater intensity, putting as much effort into the row as you can.
19-20	4-6	Cool-down: Bring the intensity of your row down to an easy level similar to that of your warm-up. Continue to row until you feel your heart rate and breathing rate return to normal.

20-Minute Intense Workouts

Jumping Rope

When you find yourself in a time crunch and you want an intense, effective cardio workout that you can do in a very short period of time, jumping rope may be the choice for you. This workout is designed to start your morning off right: 20 minutes of intense and challenging footwork that will jump-start your heart and entire body. If music motivates you, then grab your headphones and put on some upbeat music and you are on your way. Breathe deeply, and, most importantly, have a great time!

Minutes	RPE	Instruction
1-3	5	Warm-up: March in place twirling your rope in circles with one hand. Engage your abdominal muscles and stand tall.
4-6	7	Using your rope, jump lightly, alternating your right and left feet.
7-9	8-8.5	Perform a double-foot jump: Both feet take off from the ground slightly and land together. Do this for one minute. Then increase the speed of the rope and try to jump quicker during the second minute. Remember to land with your knees slightly bent.
10-11	8-8.5	Incorporate a slight jog while jumping rope, lifting your knees forward a bit with each jump. This is a slightly faster pace with increased intensity.
12-13	7.5	Move into the skipping technique, in which you alternate your feet up and down (transferring weight from one foot to the other) while the rope makes its revolution. This intensity of this interval should be slightly less than the above interval.
14-16	8.5	Transition into a moderate run with a high knee lift to increase the intensity. Be sure to bring your knee to your chest and not your chest to your knee.
17-18	8	Cross step: While in the air during the jump phase, cross your lower legs slightly and land with your legs crossed.
19-20	4-6	Cool-down: Put the rope on the floor and march in place.

20-Minute Intense Workouts

Shallow-Water Running

This intense, yet refreshing workout will leave you feeling exhilarated. Water should come to about chest to shoulder level for the best results. You will be amazed at how hard your body will have to work as you move through the water. Stay focused, breathe deeply, and commit to this quick 20-minute routine. Don't forget to wear proper footwear, outlined in chapter 5, because your feet will touch the bottom of the pool in each movement pattern.

Minutes	RPE	Instruction
1-5	3-5	Warm-up: Walk across the pool and back pumping your arms forward and back. Vary your arm pattern by swinging them from side to side. Increase the pace of your walking or begin to jog at 3 minutes to increase intensity.
6-9	7-8	Pick up the pace to a run. Run in place for one minute; then add direction by running forward and then backward. Pump your arms through the water. Make sure to come down on your heels and not on your toes.
10-13	8-8.5	Jump from one leg to the other lifting your knee as high as possible without compromising your alignment. After one minute, try to increase the pace or speed of your knee lifts.
14-18	8	Run as quickly as you can in place for one minute; then reduce your speed to that of a normal run and run forward and back for the next minute. Repeat once.
19-20	3-4	Cool-down: Walk across the pool and back while swaying your arms in front of you under the surface of the water.

Running—Speed Work

Performing this workout in the morning is ideal because your body is rested and at its highest energy level. The sprint and recovery intervals allow you to train at a higher intensity for longer periods of time while at the same time helping you increase speed and power. Recovery is essential to a good speed workout; by using it wisely, you will enhance your body's ability to take up oxygen, which in turn will greatly improve your endurance. Remember: Speed work should only be done once or twice per week, at the most. Doing speed workouts too often can lead to overtraining symptoms. You should attempt speed workouts only once you have achieved a good base level of cardiovascular endurance.

Minutes	RPE	Instruction
1-5	5	Warm-up: Jog lightly at a fairly easy effort level. Your breathing should be light; you are preparing your body here. Focus on your foot strike and body alignment.
6-9	7	Pick up the frequency of your steps here. Your breath should become more apparent. Your arms increase their swing because of the increased pace.
10-11	6	Return to an easy jog or light run—although not as light as your warm-up—for your active recovery.
12:00-12:30	9	Sprint: Run as fast as you can while maintaining good form and alignment. Measure the distance you cover during the sprint—you will try to beat it next time.
12:31-15	5	Bring it to a walk, or jog it off. This is your recovery. Feel your breath respond.
16-20	6.5-7.5	Begin to run again, returning to your original running pace. Note that you will be running at the same pace but your perceived exertion will be greater, around 7.5, because of the incomplete recovery in the last interval. Continue to jog as your body adjusts to this active recovery period and your RPE drops to 6.5.
20:00-20:30	9.5	Another sprint interval. Your goal is to travel farther than you did in the last sprint.
20:31-21	7 or lower	Bring it to a complete walk. This is another incomplete recovery—shorter than the previous one.
22-22:30	9	Last sprint. Your goal is to travel farther than you did in the previous sprint.
22:31-23:30	6.5 or less	Walk it off. This recovery is shorter than the previous one.
23:31-26	7.0	Return to an easy jog, similar to that of your first interval. This is your active recovery. Maintain good form and breathe deeply.
27-30	4-6	Cool-down: Bring it to a walk for your cool-down. Keep moving, feeling your heart rate come back down. Feel your breathing rate return to normal.

30-Minute Intense Workouts

Race Cycling—Steep Hill Climb

We're taking it to the road again this morning! Speed work is your goal. This morning you will race against yourself, trying to cover as much distance as possible in each interval. An active recovery follows before moving to the next interval. Find a fairly flat road. A slight incline or grade will not hinder the workout; it will just make it a bit more challenging during those sections. Your brain–body–breath connection is crucial here to work through each interval. Focus, push yourself to excel, and breathe deeply to keep your pace as you commit to your goal. Time to spin!

Minutes	RPE	Instruction
1-5	5	Warm-up: Begin by cycling at a speed that is easy to maintain. Focus on a smooth pedal stroke and maintaining an efficient, erect position of the torso.
6-11	7-8	Increase your pedal stroke. If necessary, increase your resistance or change gears to avoid bouncing in the saddle. At minute 8 increase your pedal stroke more to drive yourself to cover more ground.
12-13	9	Sprint for the next minute, not until you are completely breathless and out of oxygen, but until you find it hard to speak in a full sentence.
14-15	7	Reduce your speed to recover, maintaining a pace that is manageable but still feels like work. Your breath should be apparent, but you should be able to cycle with ease.
16-17	8	Increase your speed, not to a sprint level, but until you feel your heart rate increase and your muscles respond. You should feel your breath here. This is your prep for your next minute sprint.
18-19:30	9	Increase your speed to a sprint; go for it! Try to cover as much ground as possible.
19:31-21	7	Reduce your speed to recover. Slow down to a speed that is manageable and allows your breathing to ease off.
22-23	8	Increase your speed a bit and mentally prepare for the next, and final, sprint. This is your prep again.
24-25:30	9	Sprint! Give it all that you got. Just 90 seconds here—stay strong and in control. Allow your mind and body to take you there.
25:31-27	7	Active recovery: Back off and reduce your speed to recover and allow your breathing to ease off. Check your alignment.
28-30	4-6	Cool-down: Continue to reduce your speed until you are at an intensity that matches that of your warm-up. Continue to pedal until your breathing rate comes back to normal.

Treadmill

This will really put your brain–body–breath connection to the test because nearly each minute you will be monitoring your intensity. You will push yourself to increase your cardiovascular response by incorporating intervals of speed and incline changes. This is designed to be either a walking or running workout. Whichever you decide this morning, let your breathing remind you of where you are in your workout and how hard you can push yourself. Remain erect in your posture, and adapt your posture and body lean to the incline changes. The higher the incline is, the more forward your body should lean from your ankle joint. To increase your speed, increase the frequency of your steps rather than your stride.

Minutes	RPE/ Incline	Instruction
1-2:00	2-3/0	Warm-up: Start walking at a comfortable speed at which you can breathe easily enough to talk freely.
3-4	3-5/0	Begin your fitness walk or run. You should still be at an easy pace; however, your intensity should increase as you move from your easy warm-up pace to your workout pace.
5-8	5-8/.5-2	Maintain the same speed, but increase your incline to .5 percent. With each successive minute, increase your incline by .5 percent. By minute 8 you should be reaching the point of mild discomfort. Your breathing should be heavy. Maintain your form, rolling from your heel to the ball of your foot and through to the push-off. Avoid slapping your feet on the treadmill; land softly.
9	5-8/0	Decrease your incline to 0. You should feel challenged but comfortable. This is not a leisure walk or jog, just a chance to recover a bit from the last interval.
10	6-7/0	Every 20 seconds (three times) increase your speed by .1 mph or until you feel mild discomfort. Your breathing should be apparent, but you should not be breathless.
11	7-8/.5	Increase your incline to .5 percent and maintain the same pace for 60 seconds.
12	6/0	Decrease your incline and return to your base jog or fitness walk for active recovery. You should feel challenged but comfortable enough to keep the pace.
13	7-8/0	Every 15 seconds increase your speed by .1 mph. This will be challenging and should feel uncomfortable. Your breathing should be heavy here.
14	8/.5	Increase your incline and increase your speed by .5 mph and hold this for 60 seconds.

(continued)

30-Minute Intense Workouts

15	6-7/0	Decrease your incline and return to your base jog or fitness walk for active recovery. You should feel challenged but comfortable enough to keep the pace.
16	8/0	Every 10 seconds (six times), increase your speed by .1 mph. You are being challenged here and this should feel uncomfortable. Your breathing and your legs should feel a bit heavy.
17	8.5/.5	Increase your incline by .5 percent and speed by .5 mph and hold for 60 seconds. You should be breathless here!
18-21	6-7/0	Active recovery: Decrease your incline and bring your speed down to an easy run or fitness walk. Mentally prepare for your next effort interval.
22	6-7/.5	Maintain the same speed as the previous interval, but increase your incline by .5 percent. This should produce a work effort, but you should still be at a comfortable pace.
23	7.5-8/1	Maintain your speed, but increase your incline by .5 percent to 1. You should feel a slight change, but still feel you can maintain a comfortable pace.
24	8/2	Maintain your pace as you increase your incline by 1 percent. This is challenging and you should feel your breath respond.
25	8/2.5	Increase your incline by .5 percent to 2.5. Try to maintain your pace. This will feel uncomfortable. Allow your breath and body to adjust to this incline because this is where you will stay for the next few minutes.
26	7.5/2	Maintain your incline or decrease to 2 percent and increase your speed by .5 mph. This should become uncomfortable, but you can do this.
27	8-8.5/2	Maintain your incline and increase your speed about .5 mph. This is your last minute!
28-30	5-7/0	Cool-down: Decrease your incline and bring your pace down to an easy run or walk. Recover and feel your breathing respond favorably and your legs lighten up. Keep walking until your breathing rate is completely down to normal. Great job!

Treadmill—Steep Hill

This morning's goal is to cover about 2 miles (3.2 kilometers) with a workout that will build strength and endurance for your legs. The climb will get progressively steeper, so you will need to use your brain–body–breath connection to pull you through the tough portion of the climb. Remember to lean forward from your ankles as the grade gets steeper, and continue to roll from your heel to the ball of your foot and through your toes. Keep those arms pumping close to your sides, never allowing them to cross your midline. This is a tough workout that will produce results!

Minutes	RPE/ Incline	Instruction
1-5	5/0	Warm-up: Begin walking at a normal pace. Focus on your alignment: Contract your abdominal muscles, keep your shoulders down, look straight ahead, and breathe deeply. At minute 3 pick up your pace by increasing the frequency of your steps to increase the intensity.
6-10	7/1	Maintain your pace at this new incline. At minute 8, pick up your pace. You will need to adjust your body lean here a bit, leaning forward from your ankles.
11-15	8/2-2.5	Raise the incline to 2 percent. Maintain your pace at this new incline. At minute 13 raise your incline to 2.5 percent. Again, try to maintain your pace. Continue to pump your arms at your sides to stay in rhythm with your stride.
16-20	8.5/2.5-3	Remain at the pace you set in the previous interval. At minute 19, increase your incline to 3 percent. You will be breathing very hard here. Stay strong and committed.
21-24	9/3-3.5	Increase your incline to 3.5 percent, walking as quickly as you can while maintaining good form and alignment. This is the peak! It will be downhill from here. At minute 23, bring your incline down to 3 percent.
25-27	7-8.5/1-3	Maintain your pace. Stay at the 3 percent incline for the first minute; then at minute 26 reduce your incline to 2 percent, and at minute 27, to 1 percent. At your last incline change, pick up your pace a bit to keep your intensity up. Your body lean will lessen here as you become more vertical.
28-30	4-6/0	Cool-down: Walk at a leisurely pace until your breathing returns to normal.

30-Minute Intense Workouts

Stationary Bike

This workout will increase the strength and endurance in your legs while allowing you to maintain or increase your cardiovascular endurance. The workout is composed of a variety of drills used in cycling training that have been modified for work on a stationary bike. The drills will incorporate the use of the resistance option on your bike in conjunction with various position and pedal variations. Be sure to adjust your seat prior to mounting the bike.

Minutes	RPE	Instruction
1-5	3	Warm-up: Pedal at a fairly easy pace. Focus on maintaining a smooth pedal stroke and correct form.
6-8	7	Independent leg training drill: Increase the resistance until you feel your heels drop a bit. Focus on pedaling with one foot only. Keep both feet on the pedals, but concentrate on all your effort coming from one leg; the other leg is there for the ride. Keep this up for one minute, maintaining a smooth pedal stroke; then repeat with the other leg for one minute. For the final minute resume normal pedaling with equal propulsion from each stroke.
9-12	7-8	Spin-up drill: Increase your resistance, feeling your heels drop a little bit more. Maintain this resistance throughout the drill. In minute intervals, increase the speed of your pedal stroke by 5 to 10 percent. At minute 12, start to slow your pedal stroke down to where you began and recover.
13-16	8.5	Acceleration drill: Increase your resistance until you feel your hamstrings begin to work. (Slide back a bit on your saddle if you feel most of the work in your quadriceps.) Settle into a comfortable pedal stroke that you can maintain throughout the drill. Each minute, increase your resistance 5 to 10 percent; however, maintain the *same* pedal speed. This is tough because the resistance will make you want to slow your pedal strokes down. At minute 15, bring your resistance down to what it was at the beginning of the drill to give your legs some recovery time at a lower intensity.
17-19	8.5	Speed drill: Choose a resistance that allows you to pedal freely and consistently without bouncing in the saddle. Increase the rate of your pedal stroke to where your breathing and legs feel heavy but not to the point where you are breathless. The minute you feel yourself bouncing in the saddle, increase your resistance to control your pedaling. Your breathing should be hard here.
20-24	7	Active recovery: Decrease your pedal speed to allow your breath to catch up. You should still feel some resistance on the pedals.
25-28	8-8.5	Increase your resistance until you feel your hamstrings kick in more. You may want to adjust your position in the saddle to accommodate the new overload. Keep a smooth and steady pedal stroke and an erect torso.
29-30	4-6	Cool down: Reduce your resistance to the warm-up level and continue to cycle at a low level to allow your breathing to adjust and your legs to flush out. Great job!

30-Minute Intense Workouts

Elliptical Machine

This workout includes various resistance changes to push you to your limit. As the resistance increases, resist the urge to lean on the handles; instead, maintain good posture. You also may need to slow down your pedal speed. If so, keep the pedal rotation consistent throughout the interval and keep your whole foot on the pedal throughout the rotation. Remember, the elliptical machine offers a nonimpact workout, so resist the urge to bounce or bound as you increase your speed. Adding a bit more resistance may help you keep your impact level consistent.

Minutes	RPE	Instruction
1-4	5	Warm-up: Begin pedaling at a pace that is fairly easy to control and at which your breathing can remain at a normal level.
5-8	7.5	Increase your resistance until you feel a change in your breathing; maintain the same pedal rotation. Stand tall; don't bounce.
9-12	8.5	Increase your resistance until you feel your quadriceps have to push harder and your breathing becomes apparent. You may have to slow the pedal stroke down a bit here, but only enough to allow the pedals to turn smoothly while you maintain your form and alignment.
13-15	8-8.5	Decrease your resistance so you can pick up the speed a bit. Take your hands off the handles and stand tall as you continue to pedal. You may have to sit back a little on your heels to accommodate this change.
16-18	9	Increase your resistance to challenge your legs. Put your hands back on the handles and feel the change in your legs as they slow down a bit to accommodate the increasing resistance. Your breathing should be quite heavy. Don't lean forward, and don't bottom the pedal out (feeling the pedal hit the bottom and pausing before pulling it back).
19-20	8	Switch to reverse mode. Decrease your resistance to allow for a smooth pedal stroke, but increase your pedal speed. Keep your entire foot on the pedal. Continue to use the arm handles or take your hands off the handles and pedal.
21-23	8-8.5	Still in reverse mode, increase the speed of your pedal rotation. You may find it a bit easier if you sit back a bit on your heels as your drive your legs backward to maintain this action. Keep your entire foot on the pedal here, and remain vertical.
24-27	8	Switch to forward mode and continue to pedal at a resistance that allows you to maintain a comfortable pedal rotation. This is still challenging; keep your body alignment in check. After minute 25, increase your speed.
28-30	6	Cool-down: Continue to pedal while progressively decreasing your resistance. Bring it down to a level that matches your warm-up. Pedal easily with little effort as your breathing returns to normal.

30-Minute Intense Workouts

Stair Stepper

Do you feel the urge to climb this morning? This workout lets you climb to the top of a simulated mountain, then quickly descend only to turn around and go for it again. As you increase your intensity, you will feel the urge to hang onto the handles. Maintain your form by standing tall and remaining vertical throughout the workout. Make sure you allow for full range of motion rather than making quick, jerky steps that don't complete the full step cycle. Your knee joint should be fully extended with every step. Take a few deep breaths (you will need them here!) and start climbing!

Minutes	RPE	Instruction
1-5	5	Warm-up: Begin by stepping fairly easily and rhythmically. Your breathing should be fairly normal. Bring your knee toward your chest, rather than bringing your chest toward your knee.
6-12	7-9	Increase your resistance to a challenge while maintaining your speed. Each minute increase your intensity a bit. Stay steady and strong with full range of motion. Your perceived exertion at the end of this interval should be very high; you should be breathless and working very hard. The next intervals won't feel as hard as you adjust to the intensity level.
13-16	6-7	You are now simulating going downhill. Reduce your intensity and feel your breathing and legs respond. At minute 15 increase the speed of your steps, but maintain the same lighter resistance. You should be breathing comfortably at this pace.
17-23	8-8.5	Here is your second climb. Increase that intensity and climb. You may not get as breathless as you did in the last interval, because your body had had a chance to adjust, but this is still tough work. Increase your intensity every minute.
24-27	6-7	Down the stairs (or mountain) again. Reduce your intensity level. At minute 26 increase that speed again to maintain the challenge. You are still working.
28-30	4-6	Cool-down: Reduce your intensity to match that of your warm-up. Feel your breathing return to normal. Keep a tall posture.

Rowing

This rowing workout is designed to push you a bit as you work through intervals of various intensities by increasing the speed of your strokes. Rowing works every muscle in your body and leaves you feeling exhilarated. The best part is that is a nonimpact activity that enhances the coordination of your upper and lower body. This morning you will work in 10-minute intervals of alternating speeds followed by 5-minute intervals of active recovery. This complete, intense, and challenging workout will prepare you for longer rowing workouts to come. Aim for 26 to 28 SPM. Refer to chapter 5 for rowing technique tips.

Minutes	RPE	Instruction
1-5	5	Warm-up: Row for five minutes very easily, getting a feel for the technique. Aim for a stroke rate of between 24 and 28 SPM. This should be an easy row, progressively increasing in intensity to warm up your body and reinforce your alignment and technique.
6-15	7.5-8.5	Continue to row, using your entire body at a moderate yet challenging pace of 26 to 28 SPM. Begin alternating 40 seconds of harder rowing with 20 seconds of easier rowing.
16-20	7.5-8	Continue to row at a moderate yet challenging pace. This is your active recovery period for building endurance.
21-25	8-8.5	Perform another interval of 40 seconds of harder rowing followed by 20 seconds of easier rowing.
26-28	7.5-8	Continue to row at a moderate yet challenging pace, During the last minute, row with greater intensity, putting in as much effort as you can.
29-30	4-6	Cool-down: Bring the intensity of your row down to an easy level similar to that of your warm-up. Continue to row until you feel your heart rate and breathing return to normal.

30-Minute Intense Workouts

Jumping Rope

This 30-minute jump rope workout is an extended version of the 20-minute workout. Twenty minutes of jumping rope is an intense activity, and extending it to 30, 45, or 60 minutes takes a lot of endurance training. But with practice and perseverance, it can certainly be accomplished. So grab your aerobic shoes and your rope, clear some space, and you are ready to go!

Minutes	RPE	Instruction
1-3	5	Warm-up: March in place twirling your rope in circles with one hand. Engage your abdominal muscles and stand tall.
4-6	7	Using the rope, jump lightly, alternating your right and left feet.
7-9	8-8.5	Perform a double-foot jump: Both feet take off from the ground slightly and land together. Do this for one minute. Then increase the speed of the rope and try to jump quicker for the second minute. Remember to land with your knees slightly bent.
10-11	8-8.5	Incorporate a slight jog while jumping rope, lifting your knees forward a bit with each jump. This is a slightly faster pace with increased intensity.
12-13	7.5	Move into the skipping technique, in which you alternate your feet up and down (transferring weight from one foot to the other) while the rope makes its revolution. This intensity of this interval should be slightly less than the above interval.
14-16	8.5	As you continue jumping rope, transition into a moderate run with a high knee lift to increase the intensity. Be sure to bring your knee to your chest and not your chest to your knee.
17-18	8	Cross step: While in the air during the jump phase, cross your lower legs slightly and land with your legs crossed.
19-21	7	Transition back to the skipping technique, transferring your weight from one foot to the other. This is your breather.
22-25	8-8.5	Perform a side-to-side step: Alternate landing areas from left to right as you bound from one side to the other. Every 30 seconds switch from jumping with both feet from side to side to leaping from one foot to the other from side to side. Use caution as you get familiar with where the rope lands. You may want to practice this step without the rope at first.
26-28	7.5	Move to a double-foot jump.
29-30	4-6	Cool-down: For the first minute perform the alternate-foot jump; then put the rope down and continue to alternate feet without the rope pretending the rope is still in your hands. Allow your breathing to return to normal and bring yourself to a march.

Shallow-Water Running

This morning's shallow-water running workout will take you through 30 minutes of intensity challenges and a variety of actions. Because you will be performing movements that mimic running, your body will be in a vertical position the entire time. This workout will enhance your muscle tone and improve your core strength. The water should come to about chest to shoulder level for best results. In this way you can keep your arms in the water the majority of the time and make use of the resistance of the water against them. Don't forget to wear proper footwear because your feet will touch the bottom of the pool in each movement pattern. Chapter 5 has suggestions for proper choices in footwear.

Minutes	RPE	Instruction
1-5	3-5	Warm-up: Walk across the pool and back pumping your arms forward and back. Vary your arm pattern by swinging your arms from side to side. Increase the pace of your walking or begin to jog at three minutes to increase intensity.
6-9	7-8	Pick up the pace to a run. Run in place for one minute; then run forward and backward. Pump your arms through the water, creating a swinging action from the shoulder joint. Make sure to come down on your heels and not on your toes.
10-13	8-8.5	Jump from one leg to the other in place, lifting your knee as high as possible without compromising your alignment. After one minute, try to increase the speed of your knee lifts.
14-17	8	Alternate the cross-country ski motion (your legs bent and your arms moving in opposition to your legs) in place with half jumping jacks (moving only your legs in and out with your arms extended to your sides).
18-21	8	Run in place as quickly as you can for one minute; then reduce your speed to that of a normal run and run forward and back for the next minute. Repeat.
22-25	7.5	Jump from one leg to the other, lifting your knee as high as possible without compromising your alignment At minute 23 touch your opposite hand to your opposite ankle. Be sure to bring your ankle toward your hand rather than bending your torso to bring your hand toward your ankle.
26-27	8	Run in place. At minute 27, run forward and backward. Keep your arms close to your sides and your elbows bent as you pump them back and forth through the water.
28-30	3-4	Cool-down: Walk across the pool and back swaying your arms in front of you under the surface of the water. Your breathing should return to normal.

30-Minute Intense Workouts

Deep-Water Running

With deep-water running, in addition to enhancing your cardiovascular response, you gain strength in your limbs as you push and pull them through the water. What's more, your core stabilizing muscles get a tremendous workout because they have to work at maintaining your equilibrium in the water. You will need a flotation belt that can be purchased at sporting goods or swimming specialty stores or on the Internet. Maintain an erect torso throughout this workout as much as you can; you will feel your body lean a bit more forward to balance as you move through the water. You will leave feeling refreshed, invigorated, and strong. Dive in!

Minutes	RPE	Instruction
1-5	3-5	Warm-up: Begin with a progressive yet rhythmic cross-country ski movement with bent legs and arms moving in opposition to the legs, pushing and pulling through the water. At minute 3, straighten your legs and push and pull your arms more. Keep your torso upright.
6-10	6-7	Jog or run easily. Push your legs down completely through the water and pull your heels up toward your buttocks. Your arms, bent at the elbows, act as pumps at your sides. Your breath is increasing, but you should be able to maintain this pace comfortably.
11-13	7-8	Pull your knees into your chest and then press them straight back down through the water. Alternate these knee tucks with the cross-country ski movement to balance your intensity. Keep your abdominal muscles engaged.
14-16	8-8.5	Jog with high knees, sweeping your arms front and back at chest height with your palms down (sweep-outs). Focus on keeping your torso erect (your body will naturally lean a bit more forward).
17-19	8	Jog as quickly as you can, picking up your pace. Your arms, bent at the elbows, perform a quick pumping action at your sides to complement the leg action. Your breathing should become apparent here.
20-24	8-8.5	Jog or run backward. This is a challenge! Face your palms forward and push the water forward with the reverse action of your legs.
25-27	8.5-7	Perform the cross-country ski movements with your arms moving side to side across your body to pull the obliques into the action more.
28-30	3-5	Cool-down: Jog, gradually bringing down the intensity and feeling your heart rate and breathing return to normal.

45-Minute Intense Workouts

Running—Speed Work

This workout gives you more recovery time than the 30-minute running/speed work workout. Recovery is essential to a good speed workout; by using it wisely, you will enhance your body's ability to take up oxygen, which in turn will greatly improve your endurance. Your recovery is crucial to gain improvements in speed. Speed work should only be done once or twice a week, at the most. You should undertake speed workouts only once you have achieved a good base level of cardiovascular endurance.

Minutes	RPE	Instruction
1-8	5	Warm-up: Begin light jogging. Establish a pace that is comfortable and easy to maintain. Establish correct alignment.
9-12	7	Increase your speed by increasing the frequency of your steps. Your arms should be close to your sides with your elbows slightly bent. This should be a little faster than a normal jog.
13-16	6	Decrease your intensity and pace here a bit. Adjust your speed to that of a light and comfortable jog, but not as light as a warm-up. This pace is what you will return to for your active recovery.
17:00-17:45	9	Sprint: Run as hard as you can manage and still stay aerobic. Note your distance here because you will want to try to beat that in another interval.
17:46-20	5-6	Active recovery: Walk or jog lightly. Feel your breathing respond positively by backing off a bit, but you are still working here. This is *not* a cool-down pace.
21-26	7.5	Return to your original running pace. This is your endurance round. Your RPE will be more here as a result of the last sprint.
27-30	6.5	Active recovery: Go back to your light jog. Pay attention to your form here.
31-31:45	9.5	Sprint: Run as fast as you can, trying to travel farther than you did in the last sprint. You should be quite breathless here. Go for it!
31:46-33:14	6-7	Walk it off. This is an incomplete recovery. Take deep breaths here and focus for your next sprint.
33:15-34:00	9	Sprint: Again, your goal is to travel farther than you did in your last sprint.
34:01-35	6-7	Walk it off. Take deep breaths. This is a shorter recovery than the previous one.
35:01-35:45	9+	Final sprint: Don't worry about distance; just try to keep the same pace as you did in the previous sprint.
35:46-40	7	Easy jog: This is active recovery. Bring yourself down slow and steady, feeling your breathing respond and your body relax a bit.
41-45	4-6	Cool-down: Bring yourself to an easy, brisk walk. Allow your breathing rate to return to normal. You might want to take more than five minutes to cool down.

45-Minute Intense Workouts

Race Cycling

We're taking it to the road again this morning! Speed work is your goal. You will race against yourself, trying to cover as much distance as possible in each interval. You have three sprints to get through in this workout. An active recovery follows each sprint. Find a fairly flat road. A slight incline or grade will not hinder the workout; it will just make it a bit more challenging during those sections. Your brain–body–breath connection is crucial here to work through each interval. Focus, push yourself to excel, and breathe deeply to keep your pace as you commit to your goal. Time to spin!

Minutes	RPE	Instruction
1-5	5	Warm-up: Begin by cycling at a speed that is easy to maintain. Focus on a smooth pedal stroke and correct posture.
6-11	7-8	Increase your pedal stroke. If necessary, increase your resistance or change gears to avoid bouncing in the saddle. At minute 8 increase your pedal stroke more to cover more ground.
12-13	9	Sprint for the next minute. This is not an all-out sprint; just try to move quickly as though you were trying to pass someone in front of you. You shouldn't be completely breathless and out of oxygen, but you should find it hard to speak in a full sentence. Set your pace and stick to it.
14-16	7	This is an active incomplete recovery. Reduce your speed to recover from that interval, maintaining a pace that is manageable but still feels like work. Your breathing should be apparent, but you should be able to cycle with ease.
17	8	Increase your speed, not to a sprint level, but until you feel your heart rate increase and your muscles respond. You should feel your breath here.
18-19:30	9	Sprint. Go for it! Try to cover as much ground as possible. Maintain good form!
19:31-22	7	To recover, reduce your speed to a level that allows your breathing to ease off.
23	8	Increase your speed a bit and mentally prepare for the next sprint.
24-25:30	9	Sprint! Go for it! Allow your mind and body to take you there.
25:31-29	7	Active recovery: Reduce your speed to a level that allows your breathing to ease off. Feel your breath rate and your legs respond to the decrease in intensity. Check your alignment.
30-31:30	9	Sprint! This is your last sprint—so give it all you have. Imagine that a finish line is within reach, and that you have to pass one person to win. Push yourself to the edge.
31:31-35	7	Active recovery: Bring it down to an easy pedal. Catch your breath. Feel your legs relax.

| 36-41 | 8 | Endurance ride: Increase your resistance enough that you feel a need to slow your pedal stroke a bit. Stay at this resistance, find your comfort zone, and continue to pedal. At minute 39, increase your speed, keeping the same resistance. Maintain good alignment. |
| 42-45 | 4-6 | Cool-down: Continue to reduce your speed until you are at an intensity that matches that of your warm-up. Continue to pedal until your breathing rate comes back to normal. |

Treadmill

This will really put your brain–body–breath connection to the test because nearly each minute you will need to monitor your intensity. You will push yourself to increase your cardiovascular response by incorporating intervals of speed and incline changes. This is designed to be either a walking or running workout. Let your breathing remind you of where you are in your workout and how hard you can push yourself. Remain erect in your posture, and adapt your posture and body lean as the incline changes. The higher the incline is, the more forward your body will lean from your ankle joints. When increasing your speed, increase the frequency of your steps rather than your stride.

Minutes	RPE/ Incline	Instruction
1-5	2-5/0-.5	Warm-up: Walk briskly and easily, establishing your form and technique. At minute 3, pick up your pace to a fitness walk. Progressively increase your speed and intensity until you feel the need to break into a jog or run. This is still a warm-up, so your run should be at a pace you can comfortably maintain. At minute 5, increase your incline to .5 percent.
6-9	5-8/1.5-3.0	Increase your incline by 1 percent. Maintain your speed. Increase your incline .5 percent at each subsequent minute, but maintain your speed. At around an incline level of 2 percent, you should start to feel challenged and a bit uncomfortable. Your breathing should be quite apparent.
10	6/.5	This interval begins your speed work. Decrease your incline, reset your base run or fitness walk, and maintain this for the entire minute. This is a short active recovery.
11	7.5/.5	Increase your speed at 20-second intervals (three times) by .1 mph. This will feel challenging, and your breathing will respond accordingly. Maintain good form.
12	8/.5	Increase your speed by .5 mph and stay here for the complete minute. You should be breathless now.
13	6/.5	Return to your base run or walk for a quick active recovery. Recheck your form.

(continued)

14	7-8/.5	In 15-second intervals (four times) increase your speed by .1 mph.
15	8-9/.5	Increase your speed by .5 mph and hold this for the entire minute. You should be breathless. This is very challenging, but hang in there.
16	6/.5	Active recovery: Back to your normal run or fitness walk pace. Breathe deeply here and take an alignment check.
17	8/.5	In 10-second intervals (six times) increase your speed by .1 mph. It will be very challenging as you get to the fifth and sixth speed change.
18	9/.5	Increase your speed one more time, find your pace, and hold it here for 60 seconds. You will be breathless here, working *very* hard. You are at your peak.
19-22	6-8/0	This is your active recovery. Decrease your incline to 0, decrease your intensity from your last interval to a normal jog or fitness walk where you are still working enough to be challenged but can maintain a comfortable pace. At minute 20, increase your intensity a bit while still feeling comfortable.
23	6-7/1	This begins your hill jog. Time to work again! Increase your incline, but maintain your speed.
24-26	7.5-8/2-3.5	Increase your incline, but maintain your speed. Stay committed to the pace that you set before this interval change. At minute 25, increase your incline to 3 percent, maintaining your speed. At minute 26, increase the incline to 3.5 percent, keeping the same speed. This is challenging—stay focused!
27-29	8-9/3.5	This begins the hill sprint. Increase your speed by .5 mph. At minute 28, increase your speed by .5 or 1 mph. At minute 29, increase your speed again by .5 or 1 mph.
30-30:30	9/3.5	Sprint! You should be breathless—this is your peak!
30:31-40	6-8/0	For this interval you will be *base building*—that is, enhancing your normal running pace so that you eventually reach the point where you can run comfortably for an extended period of time. Decrease your incline to 0, and fall back into a normal, base jog. Catch your breath, although you are still working. At minute 33, increase your speed by .5 mph and maintain that speed. At minute 34, increase your speed again by .5 mph. Increase once more by .5 mph at minute 36. At minute 38, decrease by 1 mph. This is still challenging, but comfortable and manageable.
41-42	6-7/0	This begins your active recovery. Decrease your speed by 1 mph. This is still work, but you should feel the intensity coming down.
43-45	4-6/0	Cool-down: Decrease your speed to that of your warm-up. At minute 44 return to a normal walk as your breathing rate returns to normal.

Treadmill—Steep Hill

This morning's goal is to push your walking workout to the edge by simulating climbing a steep hill. This time we are looking to cover close to 3 miles (4.8 kilometers) with a workout that will continue to build strength and endurance in your legs. Remember to adjust your body, forward from your ankle, as the hill gets steeper, and continue to roll from your heel to the ball of your foot and through your toes. Keep those arms pumping close to your sides, never allowing them to cross your midline. This is a tough workout; you will be working hard, but you are mentally and physically prepared and ready to go.

Minutes	RPE/ Incline	Instruction
1-7	5/0	Warm-up: Begin walking at a normal pace. Set your mind to commit to this workout, visualizing the work ahead of you. Make sure you have correct form and alignment. At minute 3, walk on your heels (your body will lean forward from the ankles a little bit more here), followed at minute 4 by walking on the balls of your feet. At minute 5 return to your normal walking action, but pick up the frequency of your steps here to increase your speed.
8-12	7/1	Maintain your pace at this new incline. At minute 10, pick up your pace. You will need to lean forward here.
13-16	8/2-2.5	Maintain your pace at this new incline. At minute 14 raise your incline to 2.5 percent. Again, try to maintain your pace. Your breathing should be quite apparent here.
17-22	8.5/2.5-3	You are at your pace. At minute 21, increase your incline to 3 percent. You will be breathing very hard here. Stay strong and committed.
23-24	9/3.5	Increase your incline to 3.5 percent, walking as quickly as you can while maintaining good form and alignment. This is the edge!
25-30	8-8.5/2.5-3	Maintain your pace and reduce your incline to 3 percent. At minute 28 reduce your incline to 2.5 percent and increase your pace. You should still be breathing hard here.
31-35	7.5-8/2-3	Reduce your incline and maintain your pace. At minute 34 reduce your incline to 2 percent. Maintain your pace.
36-39	8/1.5-2	Increase your speed; your incline stays the same. At minute 37 decrease your incline to 1.5 percent. Maintain your pace. Your breath should slow down a bit, but you are still working.
40-43	7/.5-1.5	Increase your speed. At minute 42 reduce your incline .5 percent every 30 seconds until you are at .5. Your breathing and your legs should respond favorably. Stay tall!
44-45	4-6/0	Cool-down: Bring your incline down to 0 and continue to walk at a leisurely pace until your breathing returns to normal.

45-Minute Intense Workouts

Treadmill—Race Walking

The goal of this workout is to increase endurance and stamina. We will use the treadmill, but if you know of a trail in your community with a steep hill, then you can perform this workout outdoors. This workout simulates walking up a mountain road for 45 minutes maintaining a consistent pace. At the 38-minute mark, you will turn around and start to descend as your cool-down. Imagine that it's a crisp, sunny morning, and you are gazing up at the mountain. Take a deep breath and commit to this moment. You are ready to begin.

Minutes	RPE/ Incline	Instruction
1-5	5/0-.5	Warm-up: Begin walking at an easy pace and quickly move into your race walking technique. Remember, the increased walking speed requires you to place your feet in a straight line, with the inner edge of one foot landing in front of the inner edge of the other foot. At minute 3 increase your incline to .5 percent.
6-14	7-7.5/1	Increase your incline to 1 percent and continue to race walk with the intention of progressively increasing your steps.
15-17	8-8.5/2	Increase your incline to 2 percent. You are steadily increasing your climb, so increase the frequency of your steps, not your stride. Don't lose the rhythm of your hip rotation as you pick up the pace, and avoid slapping the balls of your feet on the ground.
18-20	8.5-9/2.5-3	Increase your incline again to 2.5 percent. Feel your body lean want to increase, but stay vertical and erect. Take smaller steps if necessary, but maintain your pace. Your breathing should be very apparent at this point.
21-25	8.5/3	Increase the frequency of your steps to pick up your speed about .5 mph. Resist all temptation to turn this into a jog. Maintain your technique.
26-30	9/3.5	Increase your incline again. This is the steepest part of the climb. Maintain your technique and form and remember to breathe!
31-35	8.5/3.5	There is a bit of a plateau here. Keep your pace, maintain your incline, breathe deeply, and keep going. Here is where you build your endurance.
36-39	8-9/1.5-3.5	Pick up your pace. Challenge yourself to be strong, centered, and committed. At minute 38 drop your incline to 3 percent; then 20 seconds later, to 2.5 percent; 20 seconds later, to 2 percent; and 20 second later, to 1.5 percent. Feel your breathing respond and your legs feel lighter.
40-45	5-7/0-1.5	Cool-down: Bring your incline down progressively each minute until you are at 0. As your incline decreases, decrease your speed to match that of your warm-up. Avoid running or jogging and keep walking in a narrow, straight line as your intensity decreases. Continue to walk until your breathing rate returns to normal. Great job!

Fitness and Race Walking

This morning workout is a perfect combination of fitness walking and race walking that allows you to increase your endurance and stamina levels by pushing you through intervals of increasingly higher intensity. This is designed as an outdoor workout but can easily be adapted to a treadmill if weather does not cooperate. Seek a route in a neighborhood or park that is fairly level, with some inclines. Use your brain–body–breath connection to prepare for the task at hand. As you progress through this workout, notice things around you that you find attractive to create a positive feeling that will stay with you throughout the day. You will finish with a feeling of accomplishment as you push yourself to increasing levels of improvement. Breathe deeply and focus on your form, especially when changing from one mode of walking to another. Refer to chapter 4 for descriptions of the technique related to each form of walking.

Minutes	RPE	Instruction
1-5	3-4	Warm-up: Begin with a normal walk, taking the time to set up your form and alignment. Stand tall, lift your chest, and contract your abdominal muscles.
6-8	5	Begin your fitness walk by increasing the frequency of your steps. Your breathing should become apparent here.
9-10	6	Walk on your heels, keeping your legs straight and being careful not to hyperextend your knees. There will be a slight forward lean here.
11-12	6	Pretend you are walking on a tightrope, placing one foot directly in front of the other, at the same pace as the last interval. After 30 seconds begin to increase the distance between your feet.
13-17	8-8.5	Begin your race walk and pick up the pace. Your breathing should be hard here; you should have difficulty talking to a partner.
18-21	8	Drop your pace to that of a fitness walk, continuing to walk briskly for the next three minutes. Breathe deeply as you maintain a consistent, yet quick pace.
22-27	8.5	Pick up the pace to that of a race walk; try to achieve a pace that is faster than that of your last interval of race walking. Move quickly yet efficiently, making sure that your arms do not swing across the midline of your body. Your breathing should be hard here.
28-31	8	Bring your pace back down to a fitness walk as you continue to keep a steady yet purposeful pace. Your breathing should be very apparent here, but allow you to catch up from your race walking interval.
32-37	8.5	Race walk: Pick up your pace! Try to beat the pace you worked at in the last race walk interval. Move quickly without sacrificing form and alignment. Breathe deeply and maintain your focus.

(continued)

38-41	8	Retro walking: Walk backward, making sure to glance over your shoulder to see where you are going. Try to maintain a consistent pace. Roll completely through the foot and avoid walking just on your toes.
42-45	7.5-8.5	Turn around and return to your fitness walk pace. Ensure correct alignment. Try to increase the pace here to a faster one than that of your previous fitness walk interval.
46-51	8.5-9	Pick up your pace to a race walk. You should be breathless but still remain aerobic.
52-55	7-8	Decrease your intensity to that of a fitness walk; your breathing should still be apparent, but a bit easier.
56-60	4-6	Cool-down: Continue to progressively decrease your intensity until your breathing rate returns to normal and your pace is that of a leisure walk. Allow your arms to swing naturally at your sides to match the decrease in intensity.

Running

This morning's goal is to run a 10K (6.2 miles) in 60 minutes. This workout is based on running about a 10-minute mile. If your pace is slower than that, no worries; your goal will be to cover as much ground as you can. If your pace is quicker than that (lucky you!), then your goal will be to see how much farther you can go. This is an endurance run, so you will start off at a progressive pace, conserving as much energy as possible until the final portion, but working intensely throughout the run. Pick a route that has at least a couple of inclines to help with your intensity options. This is a long workout, the longest run in this book. Many of the workouts in this chapter and chapters 7 and 8 have given you the opportunity to work up to this point. Start off slowly; use the first part of the run to prepare mentally for the work ahead. Set your alignment early and commit to your form and pace. Your breathing should be steady and rhythmic throughout, with peaks of higher intensity followed by active recovery after those incline intervals. Stay focused and committed. The result will be well worth your efforts. Let's go!

Minutes	RPE	Instruction
1-5	4-5	Warm-up: Begin with a brisk fitness walk for the first minute; then break into an easy jog. Take this time to prepare mentally. Take deep breaths and set your alignment.
6-10	6-7	Pick up the pace to a easy run by increasing the frequency of your steps. Breathe deeply and take in the moment.
11-16	7.5-8	Pick up the pace again and increase your speed. As you do, avoid pounding the pavement with your feet; try to land softly by rolling from your heel to the ball of your foot and through to the push-off.

17-22	8-8.5	Continue to run. Focus on a point about 100 yards (or meters) in the distance. Run faster as you move toward your goal, and try to maintain your pace for another 100 yards (or meters) past it. Breathe deeply, and don't get to the point where you are completely breathless.
23-25	8	Bring yourself back to your normal running pace. Catch your breath—you are approaching the halfway point soon.
26-31	8.5-9	Increase your speed as you try to cover as much ground in this five-minute interval. Your breathing should be hard here, but you don't want to be completely breathless and without oxygen.
32-36	8	Return to your normal running pace. Check your alignment: Your chest should be lifted, your stance should be vertical, and you should be looking straight ahead at the road in front of you. Your breathing should be strong here, powerful but rhythmic.
37-43	8.5-9	You are more than halfway there; it's time to pick up your pace. Run faster now without compromising your alignment. Find another point in the distance to run toward. Focus on it, trying to get there in as little time as possible. Maintain soft landings here even though you are moving faster.
44-46	8-8.5	Reduce your pace; you are backing off a bit, but this pace is still faster than your normal run. Your breathing rate will back off a bit, but you should still be breathing hard.
47-51	8.5	You are three-quarters of the way through. Take a mental note of how much ground you have covered, and let that empower you to push on. Maintain your pace: steady, strong, and powerful.
52-57	8.5-9	This is the final push. Commit yourself to your goal. Pick up the pace to a small sprint. Drive forward, increasing your speed and allowing your arms to increase their swing as well. Look straight ahead and see your goal. You are almost there. You are breathing hard but sticking to your rhythm. Go for it!
58-60	5-7	Cool-down: You did it! Back off and bring yourself to an easy run for the first minute, progressively decreasing your speed and intensity until your breathing returns to a manageable level. Continue to slow down to a fitness walk, taking more time if necessary to cool down.

60-Minute Intense Workouts

Stationary or Spin Bike

The goals of this workout are to increase the stamina and endurance in your legs as well as to gain a more positive cardiovascular response. This interval workout will allow you to train your body at higher intensities for longer periods of time so you can burn more oxygen. More oxygen consumed means more calories burned. This workout is based on a series of actual cycling drills that have been modified for work on a stationary bike. The drills will incorporate the use of the resistance option on your bike in conjunction with pedal variations. In addition, standing variations will be introduced here. Be sure to adjust your seat prior to mounting the bike. Chapter 4 reviews ways to fit yourself on a bike as well as biking technique and applications.

Minutes	RPE	Instruction
1-5	3	Warm-up: Begin pedaling at a fairly easy pace. Focus on a smooth pedal stroke with equal propulsion from each leg. Your breathing rate should be normal, and your torso should be erect.
6-9	7	Independent leg training drill: Increase the resistance until you feel your heels drop a bit. Focus on pedaling with one foot only. Keep both feet on the pedals, but concentrate on all your effort coming from one leg; the other leg is there for the ride. Keep this up for two minutes, maintaining a smooth pedal stroke; then repeat with the other leg for two minutes.
10-13	7-8	Spin-up drill: Increase your resistance, feeling your heels drop a little bit more. Maintain this resistance throughout the drill. In minute intervals, increase the speed of your pedal stroke by 5 to 10 percent. At minute 12, start to slow the pedal stroke down to where you began and recover. If you are bouncing in the saddle, increase the resistance.
14-18	8.5	Acceleration drill: Increase your resistance until you feel your hamstrings begin to work. (Slide back a bit on your saddle if you feel most of the work in your quadriceps.) Settle into a comfortable pedal stroke that you will be able to maintain throughout the drill. Each minute, increase your resistance 5 to 10 percent, but maintain the same pedal speed. This is tough because the resistance will make you want to slow your pedal stroke down. At minute 17, bring your resistance down to that of the beginning of the drill to flush out your legs.
19-22	8.5	Speed drill: Find a resistance that allows you to pedal freely and consistently without bouncing in the saddle. Increase the rate of your pedal stroke to where your breathing and legs feel heavy but not to the point where you are breathless. The minute you feel yourself bouncing in the saddle, increase your resistance to control your pedaling. Your breathing should be hard here.

23-27	7	Active recovery: Decrease your pedal speed to a speed you can control fairly easily to allow your breath catch up. You should still feel some resistance on the pedals.
28-31	8-8.5	Increase your resistance until you feel your hamstrings kick in more. You may want to adjust your position in your saddle to accommodate the new overload. Keep a smooth and steady pedal stroke and an erect torso. This is your endurance ride. You want to find a position in which you can ride comfortably at this resistance. Your breathing should be strong, but you should be able to maintain this pace.
32-35	7	Active recovery: Decrease your resistance and change to a comfortable pedal stroke. Your breathing should be calmer here, but you are still working.
36-43	8-9	Surge drill: Begin by increasing your resistance until you can no longer remain seated and feel the urge to stand. Lift your hips off the saddle, hover over the seat, and begin to climb. At minute 37, move a bit forward of your seat and drop your hips a bit as you surge by, increasing your pedal stroke as if to drive faster through your climb. Maintain this speed for about 30 seconds; then back off and recover (an incomplete recovery) in the standing position, hovering over your seat for 90 seconds. Repeat the 30-second surge again, followed by 90 minutes of active incomplete recovery two more times. You should be breathless throughout the 30-second surges, and although you are backing off on the 90-second incomplete recoveries, you will still be breathing hard.
44-46	7	Active recovery: Return to a seated position, reduce your resistance to a comfortable level, and decrease your pedal stroke. Catch your breath; however, you are still working here.
47-53	8	Increase your pedal stroke, but maintain your resistance. Try to go a bit faster to work on the spinning motion of your legs. If you find yourself bouncing in the saddle, then increase the resistance. Your breathing should be apparent here.
54-56	7	Decrease your pedal speed and maintain your resistance to flush your legs a bit. You should be at a fairly normal and comfortable spin, and your breathing should be calming down.
57-60	4-6	Cool-down: Reduce your resistance to the warm-up level and continue to cycle at a low level to allow your breathing to adjust and your legs to flush out. Great job!

60-Minute Intense Workouts

Elliptical Machine

This workout blends a series of intervals that will enhance your speed as well as endurance. It differs from other workouts in that it incorporates a variety of body positions. Because an elliptical machine mimics the motions of running, cycling, and stair stepping, you will experience a variety of postures to maximize muscular response. By tuning into your brain–body–breath connection, you can remain focused and finish feeling empowered. The morning is ideal for this workout because your body is rested and your energy stores are replenished. You are ready to take a deep breath, focus . . . Let's get started.

Minutes	RPE	Instruction
1-5	3-5	Warm-up: Begin pedaling at an easy, manageable pace. Place your entire foot on the pedal; avoid pedaling on your toes. Your heels should stay in contact with the pedal. Stand tall; don't slouch.
6-10	6-7	Increase your pedal speed as you increase your resistance. You want to pedal quickly and feel a significant difference in resistance from your warm-up. Remain upright without leaning forward.
11-14	8	Increase your resistance a bit. At minute 12, bend both knees and descend to a squatting position. Shift your weight back a bit to your heels as you assume a position that mimics that of pedaling a bicycle. You should not be bouncing on the pedals; your body remains stable and solid in the squat position. Maintain this position and continue pedaling.
15-18	8.5-9	Return to your original upright position and increase your resistance as you slow down your pedal speed to feel as though you are climbing. You will feel your muscles respond to the increased resistance as your breathing becomes heavier in response to the increased workload. The increased resistance lends itself to faulty alignment, so remain focused on your technique.
19-24	8	Active recovery: Decrease your resistance to a pedaling pace that you can maintain fairly easily so you can recover a bit.
25-30	8-8.5	Switch to reverse mode. Increase your rate of pedaling to an intensity that is equal to that of your last interval. Although the intensity is the same, your perceived exertion will be a bit higher because of the change in muscle focus. Your breathing should be apparent here.
31-35	8	Switch back to forward mode. Increase your pedal rate until you feel your breathing becoming apparent (you should not be breathless). Create a smooth pedaling action while maintaining a vertical position.
36-39	8.5-9	Bend your knees and shift your weight back slightly to your heels as you descend to a squatlike position and continue pedaling. At minute 37 increase your resistance by 1 mph and continue increasing by 1 mph with each successive minute. You should feel breathless at minute 37.

40-43	8.5	Rise to a standing position and maintain your pedal speed. Increase your pedal speed, maintaining the same resistance. Remain tall with your abdominal muscles contracted. Your breathing should be apparent.
44-47	8.5	Increase your resistance by 1 percent and continue pedaling, trying to maintain your pedal speed. Slow down a bit if necessary.
48-52	7.5-8	Active recovery: Decrease your resistance to a level that is comfortable, but workable.
53-56	8.5	Slow your pedal stroke down a bit as you increase your resistance to feel as though you are climbing. This is your last effort interval, so hang in there. You should feel your breathing become quite apparent here. Maintain good posture and technique!
57-60	5-7	Cool-down: Reduce your resistance and progressively reduce your speed, feeling your breathing respond favorably and your legs ease off as well. Feel your breathing rate quickly come back to normal.

Deep-Water Running

This workout includes a variety of drills, in addition to running, that will take your strength and endurance levels to new heights. This workout is performed with the use of a flotation belt and is designed to use progressions and elements that will challenge your core and balance while working all of the muscles in your lower body. The flotation belt forces you to stabilize your torso and enables you to experience movement patterns that not only strengthen your cardiovascular system, but also enhance your proprioception (your body's ability to sense its orientation in space and react to and protect itself against sudden forces) as well. Although your body will need to lean forward a bit, try to maintain an upright posture throughout the workout.

Minutes	RPE	Instruction
1-5	3-5	Warm-up: Begin with easy running in place. Increase your intensity, but try to remain stationary, pushing your legs down through the water from your buttocks rather than pedaling through the water.
6-10	7-8	Pick up your intensity, allowing for greater range of motion with your legs. Bring your knees up a bit higher. Move your arms from the shoulders, pushing them through the water in opposition to your legs.
11-15	8-8.5	Straddle run: Open your legs to a straddle position. By alternately lifting your knees, run in the straddle position, pushing each foot deep into the water. Be careful not to lose control of your hips behind you. To increase your intensity, increase your speed or move forward and back (or both). Your breathing should be apparent here as you increase your range of motion.

(continued)

16-20	8	Return to your normal running in place. At minute 18, increase your speed.
21-25	8-8.5	With your legs straight and your body erect, point your toes and flutter kick with your feet. Hold your hands out to your sides to stabilize your body. Keep your range of motion small and be sure to initiate the movement from your hips and ankles, not your knees. To increase your intensity, increase your speed. Breathe deeply and feel your breathing respond as you pick up your speed.
26-30	8	Return to your normal running position. At minute 28, increase your speed.
31-35	8-8.5	Reverse the basic running action. Your legs will feel as though you are riding a bicycle backward. Lift your heels and scoop water forward with the top of your feet. Your feet remain flexed. Your arms work in opposition to your legs, reaching behind your body and pushing water forward.
36-40	8	Return to your normal running position. This time try to incorporate a small movement forward and back, increasing your speed halfway through the interval. Check your form and alignment.
41-45	8.5-9	Starting from a strong vertical position, alternately lift and extend each leg forward. The leg should be bent and externally rotated at the knee. This means that as you press your leg through the water, you are leading with your inner thigh. Make sure you move only one leg at a time; the other leg remains deep beneath you for balance. While lifting your leg, reach and press your opposite hand to your ankle. Try not to bend too much from your waist; instead, lift the leg and reach forward. To increase your intensity, increase your speed.
46-49	8	Return to your normal running position. Focus here on increasing your range of motion by lifting your knees higher toward your chest (avoiding leaning forward from the waist) and then pushing your legs down through the water.
50-53	8.5	Half jacks: Starting from a feet-together, vertical position, opens your legs to a straddle position. From the widest position you are comfortable with, draw your legs back together. Focus on pushing the water away as your legs move apart, and pulling the water in as your legs come together. Aim for good range of motion, keeping your arms at the surface as stabilizers. Keep your body erect. This exercise challenges your torso stabilizers to keep a strong vertical position. To increase intensity, increase your speed.
54-57	8	Return to your normal running position. Pick up your speed here for the first 90 seconds. For the second half of the interval, reduce your speed a bit, but maintain a consistent speed that allows your breathing to respond favorably, although you are still working aerobically.
58-60	5-7	Cool-down: Continue to decrease your speed and progressively decrease your range of motion until you feel your breathing rate return to normal.

10

Recovery Workouts

In this chapter we review the elements of recovery and suggest ways you can work out during recovery. Sometimes we exhibit little traits of perfectionism: We are not content until we feel we have completed a long list of items on our to-do list for the day, for example. This perfectionism can show up in our relationship with our morning cardio workout. We may believe that we advance toward our fitness goals only when we work out day after day. The truth is, however, that unless the body has ample time to recover through rest, the risk of injury increases quite considerably. Furthermore, when you ask your body to perform intensely when your muscular systems have not had time to rest adequately, the workout is not as profitable because your muscles cannot perform at their full capacity again (American Council on Exercise 2003, 2004). This chapter describes some ways to allow the body's cardiopulmonary and muscular systems to rest while simultaneously giving those of us who feel like we absolutely *have* to work out a very different, nontraditional type of early morning cardio workout called the *recovery workout*.

Recovery workouts help your body gain more by doing *less*. A recovery workout fits into your schedule best between days of intense interval training. These workouts offer lighter-intensity options for those days when you are looking to work out less intensely, or simply to rest and recover.

The recovery workouts described in this chapter are ideal for when you are in any of the following situations:

- Scheduled to work out but feel more tired than normal
- Sore in your legs or shoulders (or both) from lack of appropriate rest
- Wanting to exercise but have not rested 24 to 48 hours from your last intense exercise session
- Feeling less energetic than normal
- For females: In the first few days of your monthly cycle, especially during heavy cycles
- Experiencing cold-like symptoms but do *not* have a flu (Avoid exercising with the flu, fever, or flu-like symptoms without consulting your medical care practitioner because your body most probably needs rest time to heal.)

Mind–Body Walking Recovery Workout

The purpose of mind–body walking is to train the brain–body–breath connection (optimal body awareness by keeping your thoughts in the present moment) during a day of recovery and relative rest. You do this by keeping a constant focus on your five senses with every foot strike against the ground. In this workout, you maintain your heart rate at a lower intensity from your more traditional workouts, for a maximum of 40 minutes. During this recovery workout, you will enjoy some slow techniques you cannot incorporate as easily into your other, more intense workouts. This workout is *not* designed to improve your fitness level, but rather to satisfy your need to move without overworking the cardiovascular system. Finally, because you are working at a lower intensity than in your other morning cardio workouts, you can dedicate time to training and improving balance, a necessary component to your overall fitness level.

For the mind–body walk, choose an area void of distractions so you can focus inwardly. Distractions include loud noises, too many other people, strong odors, irregular ground, or anything else that may keep you from maintaining a calm and comfortable walking pace. An outdoor area is ideal because the mind–body walk works best when you are engulfed in nature, surrounded by flora and fauna. Plan your workout ahead of time. If you do plan to walk outdoors, have mapped out in your head the area where you plan to go before you commence. Depending on your geographic area and weather, you may need to choose an indoor area such as a running track or treadmill. If you are walking indoors, choose the speed, time, and incline before you begin, ensuring that you have chosen an intensity below the intensity level you normally work out at.

If you decide to walk with music, choose music that is different from what you normally use in your morning cardio workouts to cue your brain, body, and breath that this workout is less intense than normal. Unlike the music that works best for your intense morning workouts, music with no regular beats per minute works best for a mind–body walk. Instrumental, New Age, mind–body, yoga, or lyrically inspirational music will help your brain, body, and breath establish this workout as distinctively different from your more intense workouts.

As always, make sure your breath is consistent and complete. For the mind–body walk, however, try to use your mouth for breathing less than you normally do during intense workouts. The first reason is that, if you are breathing heavily through your mouth, you may not be in the lower-intensity part of the exertion scale. The second reason is that you can use the nose for its original purpose, which is to bring the breath into the body as a life force through both nostrils. The third reason is that the nose allows you to capture the outdoor scents should you be fortunate enough to find yourself walking among jasmine trees in the spring, for example.

The most important part of a mind–body walk is keeping a present mind-set during every footfall. Keep your body tall and your spine extended during your walk. Your gait should be normal, with a speed that allows you to remain at a lower intensity. If you are using the recommended ranges for perceived exertion as explained on page 93, try to be below 5. To train the brain–body–breath connection, practice taking inventory of your senses, answering the following questions in rotary fashion. After you answer each question, cycle back and begin the questions again.

1. What do my eyes see? What color stands out? Do I see happiness in anything?
2. What do my ears hear? What sound stands out? Do I hear happiness in anything?
3. What does my nose smell? What smell stands out? Do I smell happiness in anything?
4. How does my breathing feel? How does my breathing alone tell me about where I am and my intensity level?
5. What does my entire body feel? What emotion stands out? What am I learning about my body during this recovery time?

Try not to get distracted by any thoughts of past or future. Remember that the purpose of the mind–body walk is to train yourself to hone your brain–body–breath awareness in our trilogy. Distracting thoughts—both feelings and judgments—are normal, such as: "What is on my agenda for the rest of the day?" "I need to start running because this low intensity is a waste of time," or, "I don't see anyone else walking." Instead of judging yourself for having such thoughts, simply acknowledge them and try to focus again on the preceding questions.

During your walk, try incorporating some of the following ideas to enhance the brain–body–breath connection.

From the Teachings of Moshe Feldenkrais Moshe Feldenkrais was an Israeli physicist who is probably best known for developing an internationally popular wellness system called the *Feldenkrais Method*. He worked for many years helping people increase the overall quality of their lives with his method, which is centered on "Awareness in Movement" lessons. A Feldenkrais lesson does not have any particular pattern of exercises. Instead, a Feldenkrais instructor helps a person develop new patterns of movement based on individual needs. One of the key tenets of a Feldenkrais awareness lesson is to help align the brain–body–breath connection by doing very small ranges of movement with the eyes closed. The result is that the person has to focus inwardly, concentrate on what small movements feel like, and translate that feeling into words to the instructor. To incorporate the teachings of Moshe Feldenkrais, begin and end your mind–body walk with a full-body scan. This means invoking the Feldenkrais principles of closing your eyes before you walk and asking yourself what the present state of feelings is around your feet, then your ankles, then your knees, and so forth, moving up your body. Repeat the full-body scan at the walk's conclusion. This practice will help you align your brain, body, and breath.

From the Chinese Discipline of Tai Chi Tai chi is a superb way to unite the physical and spiritual halves of the body. The benefits of tai chi include greater flexibility; excellent core strength and balance; improved muscle tone, breathing, and digestion; and all-around better immunity, posture, sleep, and stress management.

- **Sink the chi.** The movement called "sink the chi" is a way to stretch your back muscles and bring energy, called *chi* in Chinese, from the universe to your entire body. Stand tall and still with your feet as wide as the bony parts of your hips. Start with your arms at your sides, palms facing forward. Bring your arms overhead, keeping them just in your peripheral vision. When your hands are overhead, point your fingers toward each other without touching them (see figure 10.1*a*) and then slowly bring your arms down in front of your body (see figure 10.1*b*). At the level of your belly button, separate your hands and repeat three to five times. Practice this a few times before walking, and then try incorporating this while walking to invigorate your body and stretch your back muscles simultaneously.

- **Rooster kicks.** Incorporate rooster kicks into your mind–body walk to improve balance, tone the tops of your shoulders and quadriceps, and actively stretch your hamstrings. Slow down the pace of your walk to a slow-motion speed. Raise your right knee up to the level of your hips while keeping a slight bend in the supporting left knee (see figure 10.2*a*). Slowly extend (lengthen) your right leg, pushing the heel away from you as high as you can (see figure 10.2*b*). Without pausing, slowly flex (bend) that knee again and lower the leg, placing the foot in front of you so your body moves forward. As your leg extends and lowers, take your arms out to the sides like a bird spreading its wings. Raise your arms as you bring your leg up and straighten your knee, and then lower your arms as you lower the leg toward the floor. Maintain your breathing during the movement, and concentrate on fluid, coordinated movement. Your body should move forward at a slow pace. After three to five slow kick-like movements per side, return to your normal walking pace.

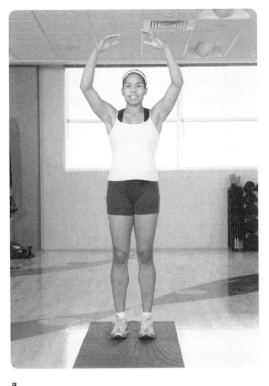 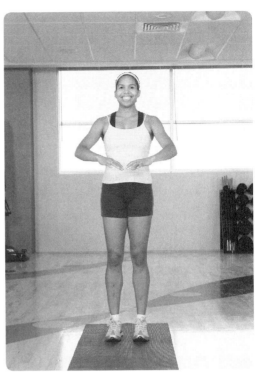

a   *b*

FIGURE 10.1   Sink the chi.

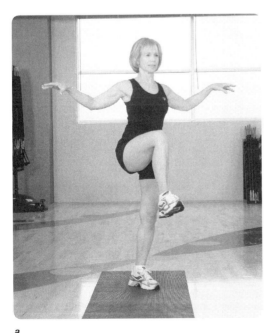 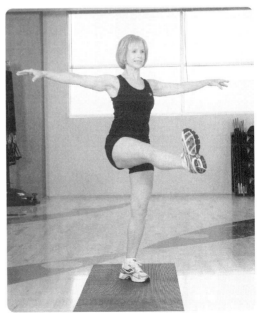

a   *b*

FIGURE 10.2   Rooster kicks.

• **Beating the drum.** Incorporate beating the drum into your mind–body walk to improve the mobility of your spine and exercise your obliques during your walk. While walking forward, let your arms gently swing to the left and right as you turn your upper body, including your head, to the left and right. The rotation to one side should last about two seconds. If possible, allow your right hand to touch your left shoulder when rotating to the left, and vice versa (see figure 10.3). Keep your spine extended without lowering your chin. Repeat to each side for approximately 30 seconds.

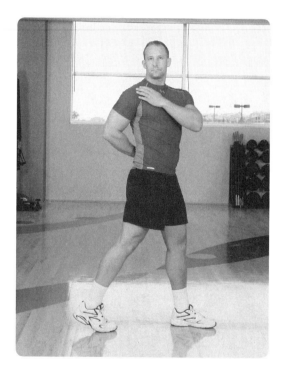

FIGURE 10.3   Beating the drum.

From the Discipline of Yoga   Incorporating some "balancing tree" yoga postures into your mind–body walk will help you stretch your back muscles and find stability and balance in everyday movements. During the middle of your walk, pause a few times to balance on one leg. Keep the supporting knee slightly bent so that you avoid placing your entire weight on one hyperextended (locked) knee. Touch the foot of the non-weight-bearing foot to the ankle, knee, or inner-thigh area of the other leg, being sure to point that bent knee to the side and not forward. Keep your arms at your side to make balancing easier (see figure 10.4a), or raise your palms overhead to touch to increase the balance challenge (see figure 10.4b) while simultaneously stretching your back muscles. An inhalation–exhalation cycle is the combined time it takes you to inhale once and exhale once. It doesn't matter how long this takes you in seconds; what matters is how aware you remain of the cycle. Hold the pose for five inhalation–exhalation cycles, or about 30 seconds,

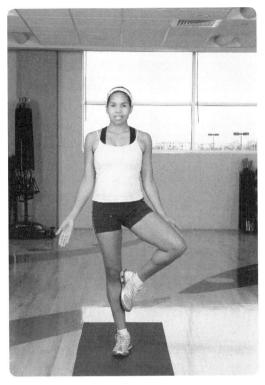
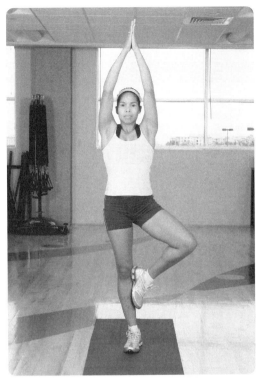

a   *b*

FIGURE 10.4   Balancing tree pose: *(a)* arms at sides; *(b)* arms reaching overhead.

focusing on looking straight ahead with a neutral neck and head. Instead of repeating to the other side immediately, try the other side after resuming your walk for a few minutes. In each mind–body recovery walk, try to have accomplished a minimum of three balancing tree poses per leg.

From the Teachings of Joseph Pilates   Joseph Pilates was born in Germany and spent most of his life sharing his ideas about proper body exercises in New York City. Unlike Moshe Feldenkrais, Pilates developed specific exercises to do on the floor or with special equipment he invented. To invoke some of Pilates' principles, try to incorporate some standing side leg kicks into your mind–body walk to train balance and exercise the side gluteal muscles, the gluteus medius. These important postural muscles really don't get much work when you run or cycle because during those activities your legs are simply moving forward and back. The standing side leg kick uses circular patterns and works the muscles of the buttocks.

As you slowly walk, raise one leg out to the side as far as you can while maintaining level hips (see figure 10.5*a*). As you lower your leg, place it in front of you (see figure 10.5*b*) so that you maintain a forward gait as you change to the other leg. Repeat for eight lifts to each side; then resume your previous gait. When you feel comfortable with the move, extend both arms out to the sides as you raise a leg, and return them to the center as you lower the leg. Breathe comfortably as you raise and lower your legs, keeping your head facing forward.

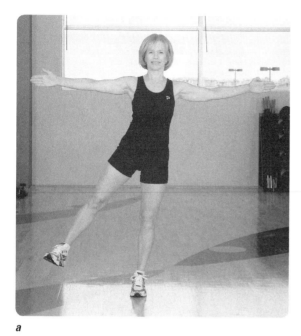

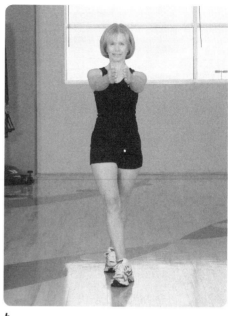

a   *b*

FIGURE 10.5   Standing side leg kick: *(a)* leg raised out to side; *(b)* leg placed in front.

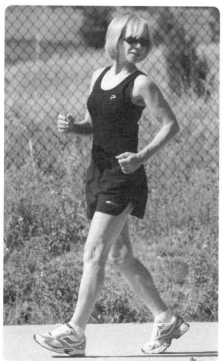

Other Mind–Body Techniques   We include the following techniques because they reinforce the brain–body–breath connection. To be successful at them, you must concentrate on the movement and breathe all during its execution. It's virtually impossible to do these correctly with a wandering mind, which is why they reinforce a mindful, meditative experience.

• **Reverse walking.** Reverse walking allows you to train all of the senses of your body to heighten their awareness and make them work together. This technique is best reserved for outdoor walking. Turn around and slowly walk backward. Speed is not important. When you look over your shoulder to see your path, do so to both sides equally, without lowering your chin as you turn (see figure 10.6). Try to walk backward for 30 seconds the first time, then for a minute, and work up to three minutes if terrain and other conditions allow.

FIGURE 10.6   Reverse walking.

• **Tightrope walking.** Tightrope walking helps the brain and body work together to improve the efficiency of your gait. This technique works well both indoors on machines and outdoors. Imagine a solid line in front of you marking your path. As you walk forward, place each foot on the imaginary line, with about 1 to 2 feet (30 to 60 centimeters) of distance between steps (see figure 10.7). As you become more comfortable with this technique, begin diminishing the space between the foot strikes, using your arms less and increasing your pace. Concentrate on maintaining even breathing cycles as you do this. Repeat for one to two minutes before resuming your normal gait.

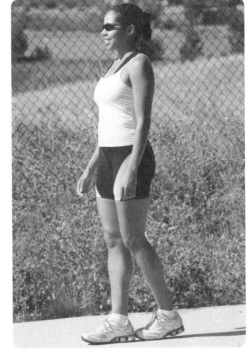

FIGURE 10.7   Tightrope walking.

• **Heel walking.** Heel walking helps to diminish muscle imbalances created from the normal plantar flexion (pointing of the foot downward) that occurs in most of your morning cardio workouts. Raise your toes so they lose contact with the ground and try to walk forward on your heels (see figure 10.8). If your pace slows, fear not. Keep the rest of your body as natural as possible, although squatting a bit as though you are making a run for the bathroom is common. Try to maintain this for at least a minute. This strengthens the muscles down the front of the leg (anterior tibialis) that often become weakened by weight-bearing cardiovascular work. If you wear shoes with high heels during your workday, these muscles are weakened even more, which is all the more reason to do heel walking.

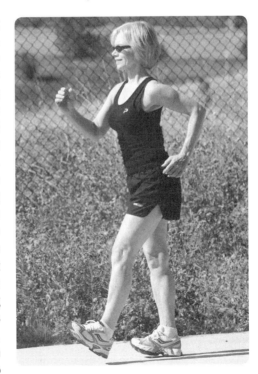

FIGURE 10.8   Heel walking.

Activity-Related Recovery Options

You can try almost any of the cardiovascular activities and workouts in this book at a lower intensity on a recovery workout day. Keep in mind that the fact that these activities are not in the mind–body recovery category specifically doesn't mean that you should relinquish the responsibility to maintain an awareness of the brain–body–breath connection. Following are some additional options for making any typical workout a recovery workout:

- Decreasing the amount of time you spend in your workout
- Decreasing the range of motion of your moving joints
- Taking away the use of your arms
- Slowing down your overall speed
- Decreasing the intensity setting of any given cardiovascular machine
- Taking a recovery ride (indoor cycling class)
- Taking a step class without the step (i.e., in a step class in which everyone else is using a platform, do the movement on the floor without the platform)
- Shortening your running distance, duration, or both
- Taking a group class catered to first-timers with a lower intensity
- Trying a new workout on a recovery day (when you are unfamiliar with a piece of equipment or type of class, your initial intensity usually is lower than it will be when you are familiar with the motor skills required of your muscles)

Keep in mind that you may have a more enjoyable experience if your recovery workout varies from your regular morning cardio workouts. The purpose of recovery is to do something different that is less than the scope of your normal workload. Recovery days are also great times to review your goals, return to the ideas in this book, and make sure you are changing the way you are taxing your heart!

Recovery and rest days also give you an ideal time to address balance. Balance means many things in fitness: mental balance, muscular balance, balance in activity choices for morning cardio workouts, balance in nutrition, and balance in strength and flexibility training. The term also signifies proprioception, which means being able to use your muscles collectively to maintain any position in space at any given moment. Proprioceptors are sensory mechanisms found in all nerve endings located in the muscles and tendons. They are responsible for relaying all information about your musculoskeletal system to your central nervous system, giving you a perception of your body's position in space. Together with muscles and tendons, they help you find balance in various positions, including standing, kneeling, and sitting. When you train balance, you are also training the way your muscles work together so that your proprioceptors become more reactive and stronger. This is important for maintaining a stable body position in every activity, reacting appropriately to unexpected changes such as when you are avoiding trips and slips, and trying new workouts safely because you are likely to remain stable. Ultimately, because your goal is to address your brain–body–breath connection in every morning cardio workout, being aware of your proprioceptors when you add balance to your workout helps you work on this trilogy. To be successful in the following exercises, you will need an alert mental state involving concentration for balance (brain), a willing bundle of muscles (body), and an awareness of even breathing (breath). On your rest day, take some time to enhance proprioception, or balance, by practicing the following:

- **Single-leg stance.** Stand on one leg while maintaining a slight bend in the supporting leg for 10 seconds (see figure 10.9). Try to increase the time you stand on one leg. To increase difficulty, bend the supporting leg more. Close your eyes to challenge your other proprioceptors more actively. Use your arms as needed: In the beginning extend your arms out to the sides (holding onto a chair or wall if necessary), and as you become familiar and proficient, practice the single-leg stance with your arms crossed in front of your chest, with your hands in your pockets, and ultimately, with your eyes closed. You will notice that your ankle muscles and other muscles "turn on" more when you close your eyes!

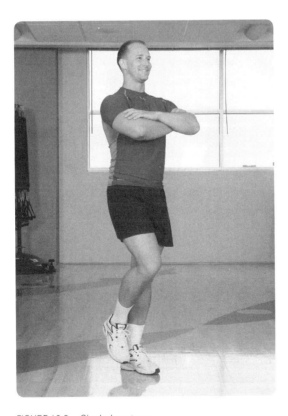

FIGURE 10.9   Single-leg stance.

• **Yoga chair pose.** With your feet and knees together, squat down as if to sit in a chair to a comfortable knee angle. Keep your arms at your sides without touching your body (see figure 10.10*a*). Concentrate on moving your buttocks (gluteals) behind you instead of letting your knees move forward. Hold the position for 10 seconds. Try to increase the time you squat here. To increase difficulty, raise one foot off the ground for 10 seconds while simultaneously raising your arms overhead without bending your elbows (see figure 10.10*b*) Repeat to the other side. Try to repeat for longer periods of time.

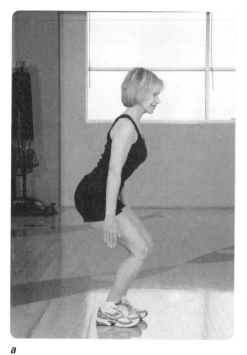 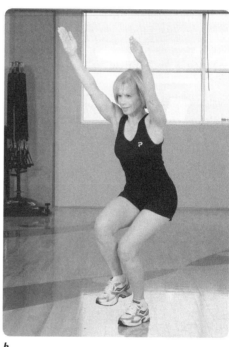

a   *b*

FIGURE 10.10   Yoga chair pose: *(a)* both legs; *(b)* one leg.

Rest and recovery are incredibly important to any fitness routine. With recovery workouts, either mind–body walking or a modified form of cardiovascular activities, the load, time, and intensity all decrease, giving you more time to train balance and address the brain–body–breath connection.

References

American College of Sports Medicine. 1998. *ACSM's resource manual for guidelines for exercise testing and prescription.* 3rd ed. Baltimore: Williams & Wilkins.

American Council on Exercise. 2004. *ACE group fitness manual.* 1st ed. San Diego: American Council on Exercise.

American Council on Exercise. 2003. *ACE personal trainer manual.* 3rd ed. San Diego: American Council on Exercise.

Biley, F.C. 2000. The effects on patient well-being of music listening as a nursing intervention: A review of the literature. *Journal of Clinical Nursing* 9 (5): 668-677.

Chek, Paul. 2004. *How to eat, move and be healthy!* Vista, CA: C.H.E.K. Institute.

Clark, N. 1997. *Nancy Clark's sports nutrition guidebook: Eating to fuel your active lifestyle.* 2nd ed. Champaign, IL: Human Kinetics.

Cook, G. 1998. *Reebok core training system.* Boston: Reebok International Ltd.

Dodd, S., R. Herb, and S. Powers. 1993. Caffeine and exercise performance: An update. *Sports Medicine* 15:14-23.

Gladwin, Laura, ed. 2003. *AFAA: Fitness theory & practice: The comprehensive resource for fitness instruction.* Sherman Oaks, CA: Aerobics and Fitness Association of America.

Hamilton, Edith. 1998. *Mythology.* New York: Time Warner Book Group.

Kravitz, L. 1994. The effects of music on exercise. *IDEA Today* 12 (9):56-61.

Kravitz, L., and J.J. Mayo. 1997. The physiological effects of aquatic exercise: A brief review. Nokomis, FL: Aquatic Exercise Association.

McArdle, W., F. Katch, and V. Katch. 1998. *Exercise physiology: Energy, nutrition and human performance.* 4th ed. Baltimore: Williams & Wilkins.

Miller, Gin. 1994. *Step Reebok: Combinations and variations 1.* Boston: Reebok International Ltd.

Reebok University. 1980. *Cycle Reebok: Foundations.* Boston: Reebok International Ltd.

Wilcox, A., A. Harford, and B. Wedel. 1985. Slim before breakfast. *Medicine & Science in Sports and Exercise* 17:2.

Wilmore, J., and D. Costill. 1990. *Training for sports activity: The physiological basis of the conditioning process.* 3rd ed. Dubuque, IA: Brown.

Yoke, Mary. 2001. *AFAA: Guide to personal fitness training.* Sherman Oaks, CA: Aerobics and Fitness Association of America.

Index

About the Authors

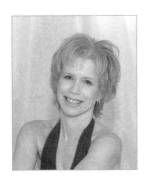

June Kahn, CPT, international fitness trainer, is the founder of June Kahn's Bodyworks, LLC, Professional Fitness and Pilates Training in Boulder, Colorado. She also serves as premier consultant and creative director for Sunshine Fitness Resources (SFResources.com), is a faculty member of SCW Fitness Education, and serves as director of Pilates for Lakeshore Athletic Clubs.

Kahn appears in numerous fitness DVDs and videos, and she is a contributing author to a number of magazines, including *Shape, Living Fit, Fitness, Fit Pregnancy,* and *Health.* Heralded by *Self* magazine as one of the Top 20 Personal Trainers in the USA, Kahn has also appeared on QVC and on Colorado television networks. A former Reebok master trainer, Kahn has been instrumental in bridging the gap between traditional Pilates and the fitness industry. She developed the Pilates Bowflex Training Program for Nautilus Health and Fitness Group and Pilates Reformer Training for Stamina Products. Kahn is a master specialist and trainer with the Aerobic and Fitness Association of America (AFAA), a master specialist/trainer and a certified health fitness instructor with the American Council on Exercise (ACE), and American College of Sports Medicine (ACSM) certified health fitness instructor. She is also certified by the Physical Mind Institute as a Pilates trainer. Kahn resides in Broomfield, Colorado.

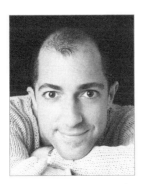

Lawrence Biscontini, MA, CNC, is group fitness manager, mind–body personal trainer, and nutritional counselor for the Golden Door Spa at Las Casitas Village in Puerto Rico. He personifies versatility in fitness and wellness education and has appeared on *Live with Regis and Kelly* and on *CNN Headline News.* In 2003, *Fitness* magazine named Biscontini one of the Top Ten USA Trainers and invited him to serve on their editorial advisory board. Cast members of *General Hospital* named Lawrence their fitness guru in *ABC Soaps in Depth* magazine.

For developing the Yo-Chi program, which fuses yoga and tai chi for land, aquatic, and stability-ball programs, Biscontini received the 2005 ECA Award from ECA World Fitness, one of the nation's leading health and fitness associations. He was also the recipient of the 2004 CanFitPro Specialty Presenter of the Year award, the 2004 IDEA Group Fitness Instructor of the Year award, and the 2002 ACE Group Fitness Instructor of the Year award. He is a certified personal trainer and group fitness instructor for land and aquatics with the ACE, AFAA, National Academy of Sports Medicine (NASM), American College of Sports Medicine (ACSM), Aquatic Exercise Association (AEA), SCW-EDU, and CanFitPro. Biscontini resides in Fajardo, Puerto Rico. For more information, visit www.findlawrence.com.

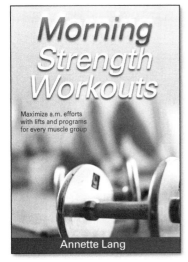
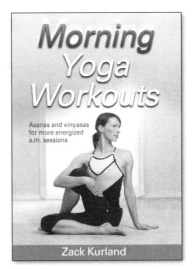
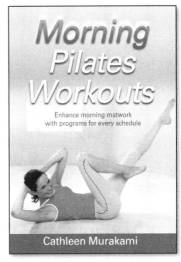